Stretching Exercises in a few min

60+

Improve mobility and reduce back and joint pain with a practical guide of easy exercises that can be done at home in just a few minutes

DOROTHY GREEN

Contents

INTRODUCTION

As we age, our bodies undergo significant changes that can limit our mobility and cause discomfort in our joints and muscles. Senior citizens, in particular, are especially susceptible to these issues, which can make it difficult to perform everyday tasks and enjoy an active lifestyle. Fortunately, there are simple stretching exercises that can help to alleviate these symptoms, improve flexibility, and enhance overall mobility. In this book, we will explore a range of stretching exercises that are specifically designed for seniors aged 60 and over. These exercises can be done in the comfort of your own home, and require only a few minutes of your time each day. We will cover a variety of techniques that can help to reduce back and joint pain, improve posture, and promote better balance and coordination. Whether you are a senior looking to stay active and healthy, or a caregiver seeking to support the health and wellbeing of a loved one, this guide will provide you with practical and effective strategies for maintaining mobility and reducing pain.

As we age, our bodies undergo significant changes that can limit our mobility and cause discomfort in our joints and muscles. Senior citizens, in particular, are especially susceptible to these issues, which can make it difficult to perform everyday tasks and enjoy an active lifestyle. Fortunately, there are simple stretching exercises that can help to alleviate these symptoms, improve flexibility, and enhance overall mobility. In this book, we will explore a range of stretching exercises that are specifically designed for seniors aged 60 and over. These exercises can be done in the comfort of your own home, and require only a few minutes of your time each day. We will cover a variety of techniques that can help to reduce back and joint pain, improve posture, and promote better balance and coordination. Whether you are a senior looking to stay active and healthy, or a caregiver seeking to support the health and wellbeing of a loved one, this guide will provide you with practical and effective strategies for maintaining mobility and reducing pain.

What is Stretching?

Stretching is an important part of any exercise program. Stretching helps improve flexibility, circulation, and joint function.

Stretching is a form of exercise that involves the lengthening of muscles. Stretches can be done both before and after physical activity, but it's particularly important to do them after an activity like running or playing soccer because it helps prevent injury by limbering up stiff muscles.

The most common types of stretches involve holding a position for several seconds at a time, then relaxing to allow blood flow back into your muscles. This allows them to recover from any contraction or tightness that may have occurred during exercise and prevents future injuries from occurring as well.

Stretching should be performed daily for optimal results!

- Stretch slowly and gently. You should feel your muscle stretching, but it shouldn't be painful. If you're feeling pain, then stop immediately and try again with less force.
- Hold each stretch for at least 20 seconds--the longer the better! It may help to count in your head while holding a stretch; this will also help prevent you from bouncing around or rushing through the exercise and risking injury.
- Stretch on both sides of your body equally so that one side doesn't become more flexible than another (which can create muscle imbalances).

Stretching helps you to relax your muscles, improve your flexibility and range of motion.

Stretching is a great way to improve your flexibility and range of motion. Stretching also helps you to relax your muscles, which can help reduce soreness after exercise. A stretching routine should include both static and dynamic stretches. Static stretches are held for 20-30 seconds at a time, while dynamic stretches involve controlled movements through the full range of motion for each muscle group being stretched.

Stretching is a warm up activity, which means that it's done before you start your workout. Stretching helps your body prepare for exercise by increasing blood flow, relaxing the muscles and improving flexibility.

If you don't stretch before working out or exercising then there are risks of injury or pain later on in the session because your muscles haven't been prepared properly for what they're about to do.

Stretching improves flexibility and range of motion.

Stretching is a form of exercise that improves flexibility and range of motion. Stretches are typically performed by slowly moving your muscles through their full range of motion in order to increase their elasticity, or ability to stretch. This can be done before or after workouts as part of your warm-up routine, or anytime throughout the day when you feel tightness in certain areas (for example: after sitting at a desk all day).

Stretching is also used as part of yoga practices and other forms of physical therapy.

Stretching can help prevent injuries.

Stretching is a great way to keep your muscles healthy and prevent injuries. If you have a sore muscle, stretching it out can help reduce the pain. You should stretch after exercising or working out because this will help your body recover faster by increasing blood flow to sore areas, which helps with healing and tissue repair.

Stretching also helps prevent injuries by reducing muscle tightness and improving flexibility in the joints where muscles attach (the tendons). Stretches should be done every day before exercising, but they can also be done at any other time during the day if needed!

Stretching can help you recover from an injury or illness.

Stretching is a good way to help you recover from an injury or illness. It can also reduce the risk of getting hurt in the future.

Stretching can make you stronger if you do it correctly and safely.

Stretching is a way to improve your flexibility and range of motion. It can help you stay healthy, prevent injuries, and increase strength. If you stretch correctly and safely, it's also possible for stretching to make you stronger!

Stretching isn't just for athletes or dancers--it's something everyone should be doing on a regular basis. When we're young and growing up our muscles are flexible enough that we don't need to stretch much (if at all). But as we get older our muscles become less flexible due to things like aging or injuries from activities like sports or dancing. Stretching helps keep the muscles loose so they don't get stiff or tight over time which could lead down the road towards arthritis later on in life if left untreated early enough now before too late when symptoms become irreversible

Stretching is important for keeping your body healthy and flexible

Stretching helps to relax tight muscles, improve circulation, reduce stress on joints and prevent injury by warming up the muscles before exercise or activity.

Stretching should be done daily as part of a program that includes proper nutrition and regular exercise. If you are not active now but want to become more active in the future, starting a stretching program now can help prepare your body for future activity by improving flexibility and strength in key areas like the lower back, hamstrings (back of thigh) quadriceps (front of thigh), calves/Achilles tendon area (lower leg), shoulders/arms etc...

Stretching is a great way to improve your flexibility and range of motion. Stretching also helps you recover faster after exercise and can even prevent injuries.

Stretching is often confused with yoga, but they're not the same thing--although stretching can be incorporated into yoga practice. There are many different types of stretching that you can do on your own or with an instructor at a gym or studio. Stretching involves gentle movements that increase blood flow throughout the body, which improves circulation and brings nutrients to muscles so they can repair themselves from exercise more quickly than if no stretch was done at all!

Why should I stretch?

Stretching is a great way to improve your flexibility and reduce the risk of injury. Stretching before exercise helps you warm up, which reduces the risk of muscle strain or tear. It also increases blood flow to the muscles, which improves their ability to perform during exercise. Stretches can be done after exercise as well--they help relax tight muscles and relieve soreness by increasing circulation through their stretching action on connective tissue (ligaments and tendons).

Stretching can reduce muscle soreness after a workout or sporting event by helping remove lactic acid from within your muscles' cells; this process is known as "lactic acid buffering." By stretching regularly over time, you will notice an increase in your flexibility level due to improved range of motion around joints like ankles, knees, hips and shoulders - all areas prone to injury when they're not properly stretched out regularly!

How do I stretch?

Stretching is a great way to stay healthy and limber, but it can be difficult to figure out how to do it effectively. Here are some tips:

- Stretch only when you are warmed up and relaxed. If you don't warm up first, your muscles are more likely to tear or strain during the stretch, which could cause serious injury!
- Always stretch slowly--don't bounce or force yourself into any position that feels uncomfortable or painful. A good rule of thumb is "no pain, no gain": if something hurts while stretching, stop doing it immediately!

Stretching can help you stay healthy and active, but there are some easy ways to make it an effective part of your workout.

Stretching is a wonderful way to stay healthy and active. It can help you avoid injury, improve your range of motion and prevent muscle fatigue. If you find yourself feeling tight or sore after a workout, stretching can help relieve those symptoms by increasing blood flow to the affected area.

Stretching doesn't just have benefits for athletes--everyone should incorporate it into their daily routine! In fact, research has shown that people who stretch regularly are less likely to experience back pain than those who don't stretch at all (or only do so occasionally).

Stretching is the act of lengthening muscle and tendons.

It's a way to prepare your body for exercise by warming up, helping prevent injuries, and improving flexibility.

The idea behind stretching is that it increases the range of motion in your joints by relaxing muscles and tendons so they can move more freely. This allows you to improve sports performance or simply feel better in your daily life.

Stretching is a type of physical conditioning that is done to improve your body's flexibility and range of motion (ROM). Stretching can be done in many different ways, including static stretching, dynamic stretching, ballistic stretching and proprioceptive neuromuscular facilitation (PNF).

Benefits of stretching include better performance, improved muscle health and decreased risk of injury.

Stretching before exercise can help you to warm up your muscles and prepare them for activity. It also improves flexibility, which is important because it allows you to move through a full range of motion without straining or tearing tendons or other connective tissues in your body.

After exercise, stretching helps to cool down the body by speeding up blood flow to reduce swelling caused by lactic acid buildup in muscles after a workout (a condition known as delayed onset muscle soreness). Finally, regular stretching is believed to improve posture while helping prevent back pain caused by tight muscles in the lower back area--and that's just one example!

Stretching involves holding a stretch for a certain amount of time in order to work the muscles further into their ROMs. Stretching is an important part of any exercise routine because it helps to prevent injuries and soreness that can occur from working out without stretching first.

Stretching should be done after your workout, when your muscles are warm and more flexible, rather than before or during your workout because stretching cold muscles can cause injury to them as well as decrease their performance during exercise.

Stretching can be done after exercise or as part of your warm-up routine. If you're stretching after exercise, make sure to cool down first by walking around and doing some light jogging in place.

When you're ready to stretch, find a comfortable position--you may want to sit on the floor or lie down if that feels best for you. Make sure that whatever position you choose does not put too much strain on the muscles being stretched; for example, if you have back problems then do not bend forward at all! In general though there are two main ways of stretching: static (holding) or dynamic (moving).

Stretching is an important part of exercise and should not be neglected. It can help prevent injuries, improve your flexibility, and even make you feel better overall.

When you stretch, it's important to hold the position for at least 30 seconds before releasing it. You should also stretch one muscle group at a time (for example: legs) so that you give each area enough attention without overstretching yourself.

Stretching is a series of movements that lengthen and extend the body. The goal of stretching is to make your muscles more flexible, which can improve your range of motion and help prevent injury.

Stretching should be done before you start exercising or playing sports, as well as after physical activity has ended. It can help you warm up for an activity and cool down afterwards--and it's important not just for athletes!

Stretching improves flexibility, circulation, and joint function.

It can also improve your balance, coordination and posture. Stretching is an active process that increases the range of motion in a particular muscle or group of muscles by applying tension to it. This may be done manually by another person or self-applied with the assistance of props such as a towel or strap (a piece of material used to stretch). There are many different types of stretches including static (where you hold the position), ballistic (low impact) and dynamic (high impact).

Stretching can be done anywhere at any time.

You can stretch anywhere, at any time. You don't need a gym or even any equipment to do it! All you need is your body and a little bit of space. Stretching is great because it helps improve flexibility, focus the mind and prepare for exercise.

Stretching can be a relaxing way to end the day.

Stretching can be a relaxing way to end the day. If you're feeling tired and sore, stretching will help you relax. You can do it right before bed or after work, for example. Stretching is also good for increasing blood flow throughout your body, which helps reduce stress and anxiety.

Stretching is an important part of any exercise program.

It helps improve flexibility, which means you can move more easily and comfortably. Stretching also reduces the risk of injury by improving muscle balance, coordination, and body awareness.

Stretching shouldn't be done before exercising because it may cause a muscle spasm (a sudden involuntary contraction). Instead, do your stretching after your workout or on days when you don't exercise at all

Stretching is a function of the nervous system that allows you to move a part of your body towards an end point and hold it. It's important for flexibility, but it also helps with balance, strength and posture.

Stretching can be done with or without the help of props like ropes or walls. Props can make it easier for some people who have difficulty balancing themselves in certain positions; however, stretching without props is fine too! Stretching doesn't have to be complicated - just take your time and do what feels good for you!

Static stretching involves holding a position for several seconds. This type of exercise is good for improving range of motion but should not be done before any other form of exercise because it can hinder performance and cause injury.

Ballistic stretching involves bouncing or jerky movements while holding a position in order to increase flexibility quickly (like when you stretch after sitting at your desk all day). Ballistic stretching is dangerous because it places stress on the muscles and tendons that could lead to injury if done improperly or often enough. Dynamic stretching is similar to ballistic but uses smooth movements instead of jerky ones; this type of activity should be used before participating in physical activity because it helps prepare your body for what's coming next without causing unnecessary stress on joints or muscles

Static stretching involves holding each stretch for 20 seconds or longer.

static stretching involves holding each stretch for 20 seconds or longer. This type of stretching is recommended for people who want to improve their flexibility and range of motion, but it's not recommended as part of an exercise routine.

Static stretches are also known as "passive," meaning they're done by an external force (such as another person) instead of by your own muscles. If you're doing static stretches on your own, make sure that you don't bounce or hold your breath while stretching--this can cause injury and may not be good for your muscles over time.

Ballistic stretching uses quick movements to force a muscle to lengthen quickly.

Ballistic stretching is a type of dynamic or active stretching that uses quick, forceful movements to force the muscle to lengthen quickly. Examples include bouncing while holding onto a wall or pulling on a towel with both hands and then letting go suddenly.

Ballistic stretching is controversial because it can cause injury if done incorrectly and may not be effective at improving range of motion in comparison with other types of stretches.

Dynamic stretching incorporates movement into your stretches to prepare your body for physical activity.

Dynamic stretching incorporates movement into your stretches to prepare your body for physical activity. Dynamic stretching is a type of active flexibility training that involves the use of controlled motions through a full range of motion, such as bending your knees while standing up from sitting position or walking up stairs.

Dynamic stretches are typically held for 10-30 seconds and repeated three times with each repetition lasting about five seconds. Dynamic stretching helps improve range of motion, reduce muscle tightness, reduce risk of injury during exercise by improving warm-up before activity and reduce muscle soreness after exercise

Know when to use different types of stretches, and how long you should hold each one!

You should be aware that there are several types of stretches and each one can be used to achieve different goals. For example, static stretching is often used before exercise and dynamic stretching after exercise. Stretches that focus on the lower body can improve flexibility in your hamstrings, while those that target the upper body may help with shoulder pain or tightness in your chest muscles.

While it's important to know when to use a specific type of stretch, it's also vital that you don't overdo it! If you're new at working out regularly then take it slow so that your muscles don't become injured by doing too much too soon (or ever).

The type of Stretching

Stretching is a simple, yet effective way to improve your flexibility and range of motion. Stretching can help you avoid injury, improve performance, and prevent soreness after exercise.

Stretching is an important part of any workout routine because it increases blood flow to muscles and helps them recover after exercise. When you stretch properly, you'll feel less soreness in your muscles after working out or playing sports--which means more time for fun activities!

There are several different types of stretching, each with its own benefits and drawbacks. Here's a breakdown of the most common types:

Static stretching

This is the most basic form of flexibility training, in which you hold a stretch for a period of time (usually 10-30 seconds). The idea behind static stretching is that it increases your range of motion by loosening tight muscles and tendons so they can move more freely. It's helpful for preventing injury but not so much for improving performance or speed.

Dynamic stretching

This type involves moving through various ranges of motion while keeping constant tension on your muscles-- for example, swinging your arms back and forth as if preparing for a race. Ballistic stretching: Ballistic movements involve bouncing or throwing yourself into stretches rather than holding them statically; this method has been shown to improve power output during exercise but may also increase risk for injury. Active Isolated Stretching (AIS): Developed by physical therapist Michael Yesses at California State University Northridge in the 1970s, AIS involves using resistance bands or other equipment to isolate specific muscle groups while moving through their full range of motion. Passive Isolated Stretching (PIS): Another technique developed by Yesses based on his work with AIS; PIS uses external forces such as gravity or another person's assistance to help relax tight muscles

Static stretching is the most common form of flexibility training. It involves holding a stretch for a period of time, usually between 30 seconds and 2 minutes. Static stretches can be performed before or after exercise, but many people choose to do them at the beginning of their workout so they don't have to worry about being tight during their workout.

Static stretches can be performed either standing up or lying down on the floor (the latter is known as "supine"). For each stretch you want to do, hold it for 30 seconds; then rest briefly before repeating three more times for a total of four repetitions per stretch. The number of repetitions will vary depending on what part of your body you're stretching--some areas require more attention than others!

Dynamic stretching is a form of active flexibility training that involves moving your body through its full range of motion, often with the help of a partner or resistance bands. Dynamic stretches are often used as warm-ups for athletic activities, but they can also be incorporated into strength training routines to improve range of motion and prevent injury.

Dynamic stretches are typically performed slowly and gently so as not to cause injury or muscle soreness later on in your workout session. Dynamic stretching should only be done after warming up with light cardio activity like walking or jogging; otherwise, you might risk pulling something!

Ballistic Stretching

Ballistic stretching is a type of dynamic stretching that involves bouncing, swinging or throwing the body into stretch positions. It's also known as active isolated stretching (AIS).

Ballistic stretches are often performed in conjunction with static stretches, which can help warm up muscles and prepare them for ballistic movements. AIS can be used at any time during your workout routine to increase blood flow to the muscles being stretched and improve flexibility.

Ballistic stretches are usually done after warming up with light cardio activity such as walking or jogging on flat ground for about five minutes. They're most effective when done before jumping rope or performing any sort of explosive movements like sprinting, jumping jacks or burpees because they get your body ready for those activities by improving range-of-motion in the joints involved in those activities (i.e., knees).

Active Stretching

Active stretching is a form of active muscle stretching that involves moving into a position and holding it for a period of time. This type of stretching can be performed by anyone at any age, but it's especially helpful for people who are new to exercise or those who want to improve their flexibility.

Active stretches are often done as part of warm-up routines before physical activity--for example, before running or playing sports--and may also be used during cool-downs after exercise. They're also sometimes used as part of an overall fitness program that includes strength training (weight lifting) and cardiovascular conditioning (cardio).

There are many different ways to perform active stretches; some examples include:

Standing quadriceps stretch: Stand with feet shoulder-width apart; bend one knee so that your foot touches the ground while keeping both knees straight; gently pull the heel toward your buttock until you feel tension in front thigh muscles; hold for 30 seconds then switch sides

Passive Stretching

Passive stretching is the most usual form of stretching. It's also known as static stretching and involves holding a stretch for 30 seconds to several minutes. Passive stretches are beneficial because they increase flexibility and reduce muscle tension, which can help prevent injury.

Passive stretches can be performed before or after exercise or any time you feel like it! Try these three simple passive stretches:

Standing quadriceps stretch - Stand with feet shoulder-width apart, toes pointing forward and knees slightly bent (do not lock). Bend forward at the hips until you feel a gentle pull in your quadriceps muscles on one side of your body; hold this position for 15 seconds before switching sides. Hamstring stretch - Lie face down on floor with legs straight out behind you; place hands under shoulders for support if needed. Chest opener - Stand with feet shoulder-width apart, knees slightly bent (don't lock). Reach both arms up over head while inhaling deeply through nose; exhale while slowly dropping arms down toward floor behind head while maintaining chest lift posture

Proprioceptive Neuromuscular Facilitation (PNF)

Proprioceptive Neuromuscular Facilitation (PNF) is relaxation of muscles to improve flexibility. This type of stretching is often used by athletes and dancers, who need to maintain their range of motion in order to perform at their best.

Proprioceptive Neuromuscular Facilitation (PNF) stretches are often used by athletes and dancers because they help increase flexibility while also improving muscle tone. These types of stretches involve contracting one muscle group while stretching another group that is not being contracted, then relaxing both muscle groups before repeating the process again with different combinations of muscles being contracted and stretched.

Tips for Stretching Safely

Stretching is a great way to improve your flexibility, but it's important not to overdo it. If you're new to stretching or have never stretched before, start with gentle stretches and gradually increase their intensity over time. Don't attempt any stretches that cause pain or discomfort--you should always feel comfortable while stretching!

Using proper form

Proper form is essential when performing any type of exercise; this includes stretching as well! Make sure that all movements are done slowly and deliberately so that they can be performed safely without risking injury or strain on the body. Also remember: if something hurts when you're doing a stretch (or any other type of exercise), stop immediately! It could mean that there's something wrong with how far back into a pose you've gone--or maybe even just one specific muscle group needs more attention than others do? Either way, listen carefully when your body tells you something isn't right because chances are pretty good there's actually something going on here...

Advantages of maintaining a flexible body

Flexibility is the ability to move your joints and muscles through their full range of motion. Flexibility is important because it helps you avoid injury, improve performance, and simply feel better.

Flexibility can be improved by stretching regularly. Stretching increases blood flow to your muscles which helps them recover faster after exercise or everyday activities like walking or running errands around town. The more flexible you are, the less likely it is that you will experience pain or soreness in those areas when they are put under pressure from activity (like running).

Physical Benefits

- Increased range of motion

- Improved posture

- Reduced risk of injury

Mental Benefits

Reduced stress. When you're in a state of flexibility, your body is more relaxed and therefore less stressed. Stress can have a negative impact on your mental health, so being flexible helps you feel calmer and happier overall.

Improved mental focus. When you're tense or rigid, it's harder to concentrate on tasks because the tension distracts you from what's happening around you (or inside). By remaining loose and limber throughout the day, however, it becomes easier for your brain cells to communicate with each other so that they can focus on whatever task at hand without being distracted by tight muscles or sore joints!

Improved sleep quality: If sleeping well is important for quality of life then increasing flexibility may be one way we can improve our chances of getting better rest each night by reducing stress levels which are known contributors towards poor slumber habits such as restless leg syndrome (RLS) which affects millions worldwide yet remains largely untreated due to lack knowledge about its causes amongst healthcare professionals - something I hope this chapter helps change!

Benefits for Athletes

Increased performance. A flexible body is more efficient, so you'll be able to move more quickly and efficiently than someone who isn't as flexible.

Improved coordination. Having better range of motion in your joints means that it's easier for your muscles to work together, which makes them more coordinated as well. This can help with everything from throwing a baseball or hitting a golf ball to playing tennis or even dancing!

Increased power output (the force generated by muscles). The same thing applies here: when the muscles are able to generate more force because they have greater range of motion and are better coordinated, this leads directly into increased power output--and all kinds of benefits like faster sprinting speeds or harder hits!

Benefits for Everyday Life

Flexibility is a key component of overall health. If you are not flexible, there are many potential problems that can arise. For example:

You may have trouble bending over to pick up something on the floor.

You might have difficulty reaching for items in high places or stretching to grab things off shelves at home or work.

You may be more likely to fall because your muscles aren't strong enough and can't support your body weight when they're stretched out too far (such as when walking down stairs).

How to Increase Flexibility

To increase flexibility, you can do any of the following:

Stretching. This is a great way to improve your flexibility and should be done before or after working out. It's also good for warming up before any activity. You can stretch by yourself or with someone else who is also trying to improve their flexibility.

Yoga and Pilates classes are great ways of improving your range of motion because they focus on stretching different parts of the body in different ways.

Foam rolling helps loosen up tight muscles so they don't get as tight again as quickly after exercise or other activities that cause stiffness in certain areas (like walking). Foam rolling also increases circulation throughout the entire body which helps reduce soreness after workouts or sports practices/games. Active isolated stretching involves holding each stretch for about 30 seconds before moving onto another one; this allows time for each muscle group being stretched (especially those around joints) so that it has better chance at relaxing into position without resistance from surrounding tissues like tendons or ligaments.

- Stretching is a great way to improve flexibility, but it's important to do it correctly. Here are some tips for stretching safely:

- Warm up first. Stretching cold muscles can cause injury, so warm up with a brisk walk or jog before stretching.

- Hold each stretch for at least 30 seconds. The longer you hold the stretch, the better chance you have of increasing your range of motion (ROM) and experiencing its benefits!

- Stretch both sides equally when doing unilateral exercises like lunges or squats; this will help prevent muscle imbalances from developing over time that could lead to pain or injury down the road if left untreated--plus if one side feels sorer than another after a workout session then that means something isn't right so don't ignore those warning signs!

Pilates Tips

Focus on your breathing. It is easy to forget to breathe properly when you are focusing on other things, but proper breathing is essential for Pilates exercises.

Practice form and alignment. The key to getting the most out of every exercise is to maintain proper form throughout each movement--this means aligning your body correctly with respect to gravity and maintaining an upright posture as much as possible (you can lean forward slightly if necessary).

Focus on proper body positioning: Make sure that all parts of your body are in alignment with one another so that they work together efficiently during an exercise; don't allow any part of yourself to be off balance or out of place!

When you practice yoga, it's important to focus on proper form. This means moving slowly and deliberately, using props for assistance if necessary. You should feel like your muscles are working to hold the pose but not straining or overstretching them. If you're having trouble holding a pose for more than a few breaths, that's a sign that your body needs to be in better alignment before attempting it again.

If one side of your body feels tighter than the other while practicing yoga poses (or even after), try placing rolled-up towels under each foot until they are both equally supported by the floor surface underneath them--this will help balance out any imbalances between sides of your body.

Chapter 1 - Stretching Preparation in Safety

Stretching is important for your body's health, but make sure you follow these tips to avoid injury.

Warm up and cool down.

To avoid injuries, you need to warm up and cool down. First, you should stretch your muscles by running in place or walking around the room. This will get blood flowing through the muscles so they're ready for action. Then, after exercising, it's important to stretch again so that they don't get too tight while they're still warm from working out.

Stretch the right muscles.

When you stretch, you want to make sure that you're stretching the right muscles. If you're not, then it's possible that your body will experience discomfort and pain. The best way to avoid this is by doing some research on which muscles are being worked out during each exercise and making sure that those are the ones being stretched in each stretch regimen before beginning any new routine or program of exercise.

Be consistent.

You can't expect to be able to stretch if you don't practice. The more often you stretch, the better your body will respond to it. Stretch every day if possible, even if only for a few minutes at first.

Once you've been doing it for a while, try increasing the number of stretches and/or the amount of time spent on each stretch every week or so until eventually it becomes part of your routine like brushing teeth or washing hands before bedtime

Cool down with static stretching.

After you've finished your workout, it's important to cool down and stretch. Cooling down allows your heart rate and breathing to return to normal so that you don't get dizzy or pass out. Stretching helps prevent soreness by increasing blood flow through the muscles and helping them relax after a workout.

Stretching should always be done after exercising because stretching cold muscles can cause injury instead of preventing it!

When you stretch, do it right!

When you stretch, do it right!

- If you're going to stretch, make sure that the stretching is done correctly and safely.
- The following tips will help:

Stretching and mobility training is an important part of any workout routine.

Stretching and mobility training is an important part of any workout routine. It's a great way to get the joints moving, prevent injury and keep your body healthy.

Whether you're stretching before a workout or after exercise, be sure to focus on the following areas:

- lower back (lumbar spine)
- hamstrings (back of thighs)
- quadriceps (front of thighs)
- upper back/shoulders

Stretching helps keep you flexible, improves your range of motion, and reduces your risk of injury.

Stretching is one of the best ways to improve your flexibility and range of motion, which can help prevent injuries. It also increases blood flow to muscles, improving circulation and reducing soreness after exercise.

You should stretch before a workout or physical activity because it allows you to reach farther, jump higher and run faster than if you don't stretch first. Stretching after exercise helps prevent muscle tightness and soreness in addition to increasing flexibility.

The most common mistake people make during stretching is not stretching enough.

When you're first starting out, it's easy to think that you've done enough when you're actually just getting started. It's important to keep in mind that in order for your muscles to become more flexible and relaxed over time, they need time on their own--without any interference from other parts of the body (like gravity). If you want a good stretch, give yourself at least 10 minutes every day or two days apart from when you do strength training exercises; this ensures that there aren't any imbalances created by overexerting certain areas while neglecting others.

Make sure you're doing the right stretches for the right reasons to avoid injury and improve performance.

There are several reasons why you might want to stretch before an athletic event. If your sport requires a lot of flexibility, stretching will help you achieve that goal. Stretching can also improve performance by increasing blood flow and circulation, which helps with muscle recovery after exercise.

However, not all stretches are created equal! If done incorrectly or too vigorously, stretching can lead to injury and decreased performance when it comes time for competition or practice. To avoid this problem:

Do not stretch cold muscles.

- Do not stretch cold muscles.
- Stretch after you have warmed up your body, which helps to increase blood flow and reduces injury risk.

Stretch only to the point of discomfort, not pain.

Stretching should be done only to the point of discomfort, not pain. If you feel pain in your muscles, stop and wait until the discomfort goes away before continuing.

You can stretch using a variety of methods: static (hold the stretch), dynamic (movement while holding the stretch), passive (assisted by another person) or active (stretching yourself). Try each method to see which feels best for you!

Warm up with a five-minute aerobic activity.

- Warm up with a five-minute aerobic activity.
- Stretch your arms, legs and back before you perform any exercises that require flexibility or strength.
- If you're going to be lifting weights, do so after warming up for at least 10 minutes (the more intense the workout, the longer the warmup).

Stretch before your activity, and then again afterward.

- Stretch before your activity, and then again afterward.

Stretching before exercise is a good idea because it helps prepare the muscles for activity. However, stretching after exercise can also be beneficial. Studies have shown that stretching after exercise may reduce muscle soreness and improve flexibility.

Stretching is important for your body's health, but make sure you follow these tips to avoid injury.

Now that you know the importance of stretching, it's time to get started on your routine. Make sure you follow these tips to avoid injury:

- Warm up before stretching. If you're going to be doing any strenuous activity, like running or playing sports, warm up beforehand so that your muscles are loose and ready for action.

- Stretch after exercise as well as before it-- helps prevent injuries by making sure that your muscles are flexible enough for whatever activity comes next!

The purpose of stretching

Stretching is an important part of any workout routine. It prepares your muscles for physical activity and helps prevent injury. Stretching also improves flexibility, which can help with posture and balance, as well as coordination and speed of movement.

Stretching is most effective when done regularly before exercise or sports activities that require strength and flexibility, such as yoga or martial arts training. The more often you stretch, the better results you'll see over time!

How to prepare for stretching

To prepare for stretching, you should:

- Stretch regularly. Stretching is beneficial to your body and mind, but it is not something that happens overnight. You need to stretch consistently over time in order to see results--at least once or twice a week! Try doing some simple stretches before bed every night, or even while watching TV in the evening (it's easy). You can also try some more advanced poses if you're feeling up for it after working out at the gym or during yoga class.

- Stay hydrated throughout the day by drinking plenty of water or herbal tea instead of sodas/coffees/alcoholic beverages (these will dehydrate you). This will make sure that your muscles stay loose and flexible so they don't get stiff when they're being stretched out later on down south there by yourself without anyone else around except maybe one person who isn't really paying attention anyway because he has his own stuff going on too much right now trying hard not think about anything else besides getting through this moment without falling apart completely

Which exercises are best?

The best exercises are those that you can do without equipment, as they're more likely to be available in an emergency. You'll also want to make sure that any stretches you do are safe for your body and don't cause injury.

Stretching is an important part of a fit body.

Stretching is an important part of a fit body. Stretching your muscles helps them to relax and lengthen, which makes it easier to move around in your daily life. You should stretch before you exercise or play sports, but you can also stretch after you exercise if you feel soreness in one or more areas of your body.

Stretching helps prevent injuries by improving flexibility and keeping muscles loose so they aren't as likely to tear during physical activity (like running). Stretching also relaxes tight muscles that may be causing discomfort or pain while also increasing blood flow through the joints--which helps improve circulation throughout the entire body!

Stretching is a great way to prepare your body for any physical activity, especially if it's something you haven't done before. Stretching helps improve flexibility and range of motion (ROM).

- Increased ROM can lead to greater muscle power, speed, and agility.
- Increased ROM may also help prevent injury by reducing the risk of muscle strain or tear during physical activity.
- Warm up. It is important to warm up your muscles before stretching, as this will reduce the risk of injury.
- Stretch properly. When you're ready for your workout, focus on doing each stretch with control and precision: Don't bounce or hold a stretch too long--just until you feel the muscle relax enough that it's comfortable to move farther into the stretch without pain (which may be different from person to person).

Stretching preparation

To ensure you are ready to stretch, please follow these steps:

- Make sure you have enough room to fully extend your arms and legs. If not, consider moving away from any walls or other objects that might get in the way of your stretching.

- Stand tall with feet hip-width apart, knees slightly bent and shoulders relaxed. Inhale deeply through your nose as you raise both arms above head with palms facing forward (or holding onto something for support if needed). Take two long deep breaths here before continuing on with this exercise; these will help loosen up muscles and prepare them for stretching movements later on in class!

Stretching and safety

Stretching is an important aspect of preparation for any sport. It can help prevent injury, improve performance and make you feel better.

However, stretching should not be done without supervision or guidance from a trained professional. It's important that you know what stretches are appropriate for the activity you're doing, so be sure to consult with someone who knows the correct way to stretch before performing any type of flexibility exercises on your own.

If you stretch yourself too far, you risk tearing the muscle.

Stretching yourself too far can be dangerous. You may tear the muscle or cause it to become strained, which will make it difficult for you to move and perform tasks.

Stretching yourself too far also puts excessive pressure on your joints and ligaments, making them more susceptible to injury.

You should try to avoid overstretching a muscle when you're preparing to lift weights.

Stretching is an important part of any workout routine, but it's important to avoid overstretching a muscle when you're preparing to lift weights. If you are stretching before your workout and feel pain in the area being stretched (or even just soreness), it could be a sign that the muscle is already tight and needs more time to relax before being stretched again. Instead of stretching too far, try doing some light cardio or walking around on the treadmill before starting your weightlifting routine. This will help loosen up those muscles so they don't get injured during exercise!

Stretching your muscles allows them to be flexible and strong, which means that you will be able to safely work out.

Stretching also helps prevent injury by improving the range of motion in your joints. When you stretch a muscle, it becomes longer and more elastic, or able to stretch further than before. This gives you better control over your movements as well as reducing the risk of tearing or straining tendons during exercise routines.

When stretching, it is important to make sure that you are not overdoing it.

When stretching, it is important to remember that you should not overdo it. If you push too hard and cause pain in your muscles, then you are doing more harm than good. You can avoid this by warming up with some light cardio activity before starting your stretching routine. This will get the blood flowing through your body and help loosen up tight muscles so they are ready for stretching when it comes time for that part of the workout.

If you want more information on how best to prepare yourself physically before beginning a yoga routine or any other type of exercise program at home or in class (or if you simply want some basic information about what exactly stretching does), check out our chapter "Stretching Preparation: What Should I Know?"

You should start slowly when stretching and increase the distance gradually as you go along.

Stretching preparation is important for all of your stretching exercises. You should start slowly when stretching and increase the distance gradually as you go along.

- Warm up by walking or jogging in place for five minutes, then do some light stretches to prepare your muscles for more strenuous activity.
- Stretch each muscle group fully, but don't overdo it--a slow stretch is better than a fast one.

If you feel pain or discomfort as you are stretching, then it is time to stop and let your muscles rest for a while before continuing.

If the pain continues after resting, it could be an indication that you have overdone it and should seek medical advice if necessary.

As a beginner, you may not be able to do many repetitions of a given exercise. Don't worry about it; take your time and build up your strength gradually.

- Always warm up before lifting weights. Warming up helps prevent injury by increasing blood flow and joint flexibility, which allows you to lift more weight safely with less risk of injury. You should also cool down after exercising by slowly lowering the weight back down again and stretching gently for 10-15 seconds per muscle group (for example: stretching arms overhead).

Choose a safe and comfortable place to stretch.

- Find a quiet place where you won't be interrupted by children or pets, or outside in the yard.

- Avoid areas with uneven surfaces that could cause you to fall if you lose your balance while stretching.

Perform warm-up exercises before stretching.

Warm-up exercises are an essential part of any stretching routine. They prepare the body for the activity that follows and help prevent injury, especially when it comes to stretching. Many people think that warming up means simply doing a few jumping jacks or taking a brisk walk around the block, but there are many other ways you can warm up your muscles before stretching if you're looking for something more comprehensive.

One way is by performing dynamic stretches--these involve moving parts of your body in different directions while holding certain positions (like lunges). These types of movements get blood flowing through all areas of your body, including those that are going to be stretched later on! Another option is ballistic stretches: these involve bouncing at high speeds while holding poses like runner's lunge or hurdler's stretch; they're known as ballistic because they require quick movements without much control over where one lands after each bounce (similarly to how one might throw a ball).

Breathe normally while you're stretching.

- Breathe normally while you're stretching.

- Do not hold your breath. If you do, your muscles will tighten and make it harder to stretch them, which can lead to injury.

A little preparation goes a long way toward making your stretches safe and effective

Here are some tips for stretching safely and effectively:

- Warm up your muscles by doing some gentle movement before you stretch. This can include walking or jogging in place, marching in place, or doing jumping jacks.

- Do not stretch when you are tired or stressed out--wait until after you've cooled down and relaxed a little bit before stretching out again!

- Stretch gently--you should feel the stretch in the muscle being stretched, but don't overdo it! You should be able to hold each stretch for 30 seconds without pain or discomfort; if something hurts (or if there's no sensation), stop immediately and find another way to stretch that area instead!

Stretching is a lot like working out.

The more you stretch, the looser and more flexible your muscles become. If you don't stretch regularly, your muscles can become tight and inflexible over time--and that can lead to injuries. So, if you're not doing any kind of regular exercise yet (or even if you are), start with some basic stretches to get started on this important part of staying safe in climbing!

You need to prepare your body for stretching in order to see the best results.

In order to reap the benefits of stretching, you need to prepare your body for it. This means warming up before stretching, stretching slowly and gently, and holding each stretch for at least 30 seconds.

WARNING: Stretching can be dangerous if done incorrectly or without preparation. If you have any medical conditions or injuries that prevent you from stretching safely, please consult a doctor before attempting any form of physical activity!

Stretching is not just about flexibility.

- Stretching is not just about flexibility.
- Stretching can help you to avoid injuries, improve your performance and reduce muscle soreness. Stretching also enhances blood flow, which helps you recover faster after exercise.
- When you stretch a muscle, it increases its ability to relax and lengthen. This allows for greater flexibility in the joints above or below that particular muscle group (for example: stretching your quadriceps will improve your hamstring flexibility).

If you're feeling stiff, it's time to stretch. Stretching is a great way to increase your flexibility and reduce muscle tension. However, stretching incorrectly can cause injury or pain. Follow these steps to ensure that you are doing it safely:

- Stretch only after warming up with some light cardio exercise (such as walking) for 5-10 minutes. This will increase blood flow through your muscles and make them more pliable for stretching.

- Stretch in an area where there is no chance of falling over; it's important that your balance be steady while attempting any form of static stretching (holding one position for an extended period).
- Use proper posture when performing each stretch; keep your back straight and chest lifted throughout each movement so that you don't strain any part of the body unnecessarily due to poor alignment during exercise!

Stretching is an important part of a healthy life, and you should do it right!

Stretching is an important part of a healthy life, and you should do it right! If you're stretching for the first time, or even if you've been at it for a while, there are some things to keep in mind. Here are some tips to help keep your stretches safe:

- Stretch regularly. This is probably obvious, but if you don't stretch regularly--and especially if this is new to you-- could hurt yourself by doing too much too soon or not stretching enough overall. Make sure that every stretch feels comfortable before moving on to another muscle group or exercise.
- Avoid overstretching. Overstretching can lead not only to injury but also loss of range-of-motion due to muscle tightness; therefore, avoid going beyond what feels comfortable when stretching under any circumstances!

Stretching is essential before training to reduce the risk of injury.

Stretching is essential before training to reduce the risk of injury. While stretching, you should feel a slight pull in your muscles but not pain. If you feel pain, stop stretching immediately and consult with a doctor or physical therapist if necessary.

Stretching helps prevent injuries by reducing muscle tension before exercise and increasing blood flow to the muscles, which delivers oxygen and nutrients needed for activity. Stretching also increases flexibility by lengthening muscle fibers by breaking down connective tissue (scar tissue) that has formed over time due to injury or repetitive use without proper recovery periods between workouts/races/exercises etc...

Stretching actively increases your range of motion, but passively decreases it.

- Stretching actively increases your range of motion, but passively decreases it.

- When you stretch, the muscle fibers are pulled apart and lengthened. This causes the muscle to become slightly weaker as it gets longer and thinner; this is called "negative tension". When we stretch a muscle over time (as in yoga), we are actually training our muscles to be able to stretch more easily than before. This is because there is less resistance from within the tissue itself when we extend them at an angle away from their normal resting length--so they become easier for us to do so!

Static stretching should be held for no more than 30 seconds.

The most important thing to remember about static stretching is that it should be held for no more than 30 seconds. Any longer than that and you risk damaging your muscles, which can lead to injury in the long run.

In addition, static stretching shouldn't be performed before or after a workout or competition because it will interfere with muscle strength and power development. Instead, consider using dynamic warm-up movements like jumping jacks or squats as an alternative method of preparing your body for exercise--this will help activate your muscles without compromising their function or increasing the risk of injury later on when performing more intense activities such as weightlifting or running (2).

Hold stretches in the same position throughout their duration.

Hold stretches in the same position throughout their duration.

- For example, if you are doing a quad stretch, keep your leg straight throughout the stretch and do not bend or flex it at all. The only exception is when you need to move to another position that requires a different body part (such as switching from stretching one side of your quadriceps to stretching the other side).

You can use stretching to improve your athletic performance and reduce an injury risk

You can use stretching to improve your athletic performance and reduce an injury risk.

Stretching is a great way to prepare for exercise, especially if you're new to it. Stretching helps increase flexibility in muscles and tendons, which can help prevent injury during workouts or sports. Stretching also helps improve coordination between the brain and muscles so that movements are smoother and more precise--this can translate into better results in sports!

Always prepare your muscle and joints before stretching by warming up.

Warm up before stretching.

- Do some light cardio, such as walking or jogging.
- Perform a few dynamic warm-up exercises to prepare the body for physical activity, including jumping jacks and arm circles (or shoulder rolls).

Stretch slowly and carefully, not fast and hard.

- Stretch slowly and carefully, not fast and hard.
- Do not bounce.
- Breathe normally while stretching, do not hold your breath.

Focus on the muscles that are being stretched.

- Focus on the muscles that are being stretched.

When you're stretching, it's important to concentrate on the muscles that are being stretched. If you focus on other parts of your body (such as your back or neck), then this could cause injury or discomfort.

- Maintain good posture while stretching.

Stretching requires good posture so that you don't strain any joints unnecessarily; this means keeping your head up and shoulders back while doing so, as well as using proper breathing techniques throughout each stretch session

Do not bounce while you are stretching.

Bouncing is bad for your joints and can cause injury. The goal of stretching is to slowly increase your range of motion, so you don't want to bounce or otherwise force your muscles into a stretch they're not ready for. Instead, gently move into the stretch until you feel the muscles relax and become pliable before holding the position for at least 30 seconds (more is better).

Avoid overstretching, which may cause tears in your muscles and tendons.

To avoid overstretching, which may cause tears in your muscles and tendons:

- Warm up with light stretches. Stretching before an activity is important for warming up muscles, but be careful not to overdo it. If you're going for a run or bike ride, start by walking at first and then gradually increase your speed as your body warms up.

- Hold each stretch for at least 30 seconds--and no more than 60 seconds--to prevent injury from overextension of joints or muscles (when they are stretched beyond their normal range).

If you follow these tips for preparing for a stretch, you can avoid injury when you do it.

If you follow these tips for preparing for a stretch, you can avoid injury when you do it.

- Get warmed up first. Stretching cold muscles can cause injury and pain, so it's important to warm up before stretching by doing some light cardio or other exercises that get your blood flowing.

- Know how far to go with each stretch. Don't push past the point where it feels uncomfortable--you should feel some tension in the muscle being stretched but not pain or tearing sensation! It's better to hold a stretch for 20 seconds than 10 seconds if that means avoiding injury!

- Move slowly through each position of the exercise; don't bounce around quickly from one position to another because this could cause injury as well (especially if someone else is helping hold down your limbs).

Chapter 2 – Warm-up exercises

Exercise is an important part of life, but sometimes we forget how to warm up. For some people, stretching seems like a waste of time; they just want to get right into their workout. But if you don't warm up properly before exercise or physical activity, you can actually cause more harm than good! A proper warm-up includes movement and flexibility exercises that help loosen muscles and joints so they're ready for the demands placed on them during exercise.

Warm-up exercises

Warm-up exercises are a series of movements that prepare the body for activity. The goal is to warm up muscle tissues and improve blood flow, which helps to prevent injury. Because the muscles are less able to perform at peak levels during a cold state, warming up reduces the risk of strains and pulls.

It's important that you start off slowly when performing your warm-up exercises; they should be done slowly enough so that they do not cause pain or discomfort in any part of your body.

Stretching

Stretching is an important part of any exercise routine. It helps to prevent injury, and it also increases flexibility, which can be useful in your workout. Stretches should be performed at least once a day, but it's best if you include them in your warm-up routine before each workout session as well. You should stretch every muscle group that will be used during the exercise session--this includes any major muscle groups such as those in the legs, arms and back.

You should stretch until feeling slight tension on the muscle being stretched; this means that it may take some time for each stretch to become effective. Do not bounce during stretching exercises or allow yourself to be distracted by other people around you who might do so; this could cause injury!

Exercise

This warm-up exercise is called the "cat stretch."

To perform this exercise, begin by sitting on the floor with both legs straight out in front of you. Bend forward and place both hands on the floor in front of your feet. Bring one leg up toward your chest while keeping the other straight out behind you; then switch legs and repeat for 10 repetitions per side (5 each time).

Benefits: The cat stretch helps to loosen up muscles before they're used during a workout, so they can move more freely during exercise routines or sports activities. It also stretches out hips, hamstrings and calves--all areas that get tight when we sit too much throughout our day!

How often?: You should perform 1-2 sets of 5 reps every day as part of an overall warm up routine before working out at home!

Exercise 2

Warm up exercises are an important part of your workout routine. They help you get loose and ready for the main part of your exercise, which is why they should be the first thing you do before working out.

- Do jumping jacks for 1 minute to get your heart rate up and blood flowing through your body.
- Stand with feet shoulder-width apart and raise both arms above head, palms facing forward (as if holding a basketball). Bend forward at waist until hands touch floor in front of right foot; return to standing position by raising left leg behind right knee then stepping out with left foot onto floor behind right toe while simultaneously lowering arms back down toward chest level - repeat on opposite side (this is one repetition). Do 10 reps per side before continuing onto next warmup activity

Cool down.

Cool down exercises are a series of movements that help the body recover from activity. They should take place after exercise has ended and before you go home, so that your muscles have time to cool down.

Cool down exercises are important for preventing injuries, and for reducing muscle soreness. They also help flush out lactic acid (a byproduct of energy production) from your muscles so that they don't stiffen up while you're sitting around doing nothing!

If you have not been doing any cool down exercises before now, try starting with one or two of these:

Warm-up exercises are a series of movements that prepare the body for activity.

. The goal is to warm up muscle tissues and improve blood flow, which helps to prevent injury. Because the muscles are less able to perform at peak levels during a cold state, warming up reduces the risk of strains and pulls.

The goal of a warmup exercise is to warm up muscle tissues and improve blood flow, which helps to prevent injury. A good warm up will also prepare your body for the activity that's about to follow.

If you're not sure how much time you should spend warming up before a workout, it might help if you think about what kind of activity you're doing: If it's something like running or biking (or any cardio), then about 10 minutes should be sufficient; if it's strength training or resistance training (like lifting weights), then 15-20 minutes would be better; but if it's yoga or Pilates and involves stretching as well...30 minutes might be best!

Warming up reduces the risk of strains and pulls.

When you start exercising, your body is not at its peak level of performance. Your muscles are less able to perform at peak levels during a cold state, which means that warming up reduces the risk of strains and pulls.

All activities require a warm-up because no one knows what their body will need before they begin an exercise routine.

Warming up before exercise is important because no one knows what their body will need before they begin an exercise routine. A warm-up should be done at least five minutes before your main workout and should consist of light aerobic activity and low-impact stretching.

- Aerobic Activity: This can include jogging, jumping rope or riding a stationary bike for about five minutes. It's best to start with this step because it helps increase blood flow throughout the body, which reduces risk of injury during more intense activities later on in your workout session.
- Stretching: Static stretches are best performed after aerobic activity; dynamic stretches should come first if possible (see below). Static stretches involve holding each stretch for 30 seconds while breathing deeply through pursed lips until you feel a slight pull from the muscle being stretched--but not pain! Be sure not to overstretch yourself because this could result into injury or soreness later on in the day when you're at

work or school instead of working out again after taking some time off due to being too sore from doing too many static stretches earlier that morning

A proper warm-up can reduce the likelihood of injury during exercise.

A proper warm-up can reduce the likelihood of injury during exercise. Warm-up exercises are a series of movements that prepare the body for activity, increase blood flow and improve muscle elasticity. The goal is to warm up muscle tissues and improve blood flow, which helps to prevent injury by improving flexibility and reducing the risk of strains or tears in muscles or tendons.

Warm-up exercises are important before any physical activity, especially if you're not used to doing that type of exercise or if it's been a while since your last workout. A warm-up helps loosen your muscles and get them ready for the more intense activity ahead.

The best types of warm-ups vary depending on what kind of activity you're going to do:

- For sports, try running around the field or court several times at an easy pace before starting playtime. If possible, do some stretches while waiting for other players' turns in line (like when waiting for a serve).

- For running races like 5Ks or marathons: Walk briskly for 5 minutes before starting out at an easy jog pace until halfway through the race distance (about 1 mile), then gradually increase speed toward faster running speeds until finishing line is reached!

Before you begin the exercises, there are a few things you need to know:

- Stretching is an important part of any workout routine. It helps prevent injury by increasing flexibility and improving your range of motion.

- The heel raise exercise is one way to increase the flexibility in your ankles and Achilles tendons. To do this exercise, stand on the edge of your toes for about five seconds before lowering yourself back down onto flat feet again; repeat this movement 10 times or more if possible without discomfort.

Downward Dog

Downward Dog is a great exercise for stretching and strengthening the spine, back, arms, legs and shoulders. It also helps to improve posture as well as balance.

Downward Dog can be done after you have warmed up your body with some light cardio such as jogging in place or jumping jacks. This will help prevent injury when doing this stretch because it will be easier on your joints if they are already warmed up when starting downward dog pose (see below).

Side Plank

Side Plank with Arm and Leg Lift

This exercise is a fantastic way to strengthen your core while improving balance. Lie on your side, propped up by your forearm and top knee. Lift both arms up, then lower them down while keeping the rest of your body still. Repeat 10 times per side before switching sides and repeating another 10 reps for each side again (20 total).

Side Plank with Arm and Leg Twist

This variation requires less strength than the previous one but will still give you an intense workout! Instead of lifting just one arm at a time like in #1 above, try lifting both arms together as well as twisting from side-to-side for an extra challenge on those obliques!

Lunge Pose

Lunges are a great way to strengthen your legs and butt, but they can also be good for your core muscles. Lunges can be performed with weights, dumbbells or even a barbell if you want to take it up a notch!

There are three main types of lunges: forward, reverse and lateral. In all cases you will start by standing upright with feet hip-width apart (or wider) then step forward into the lunge position before returning to starting position

Chapter 3 – Morning Stretching Exercises

Let us face it: the morning is not a good time for me. I'm groggy, my brain isn't working full speed yet and sometimes I don't even remember where I am. Which means that stretching? Not happening when you wake up! But if you are like me, then you know that stretching is an important part of staying in shape. And although some people just hop out of bed and go about their day without even realizing how stiff they are, others prefer to do morning stretching exercises before they start moving around too much. If this sounds like you (and let's be honest here—it probably does), then read on! Here are some easy ways to make sure your body stays limber throughout the day:

Morning stretching exercises range in length from 5-10 minutes and are focused on flexibility, strength, and balance.

The first step is to start with a warm up. This can be as simple as walking around the house or doing some jumping jacks. Next comes stretching your arms, legs, chest and back by reaching for the sky with each arm while keeping your feet flat on the ground. Then move onto pelvic tilts which helps with core strength by gently tightening your abdominal muscles then relaxing them again for about 10 repetitions (1 set). Next is downward facing dog pose where you bend forward at the hips while keeping both legs straight; this helps stretch out your hamstrings as well as build core strength because it requires lifting one leg off of its respective side while also holding onto something sturdy to keep yourself balanced during this exercise (2 sets). Finally wind down by lying flat on your back with knees bent up towards chest level before repeating everything all over again!

Stand with your feet hip-width apart.

Stand with your feet hip-width apart and place a hand on each knee. Lift one leg up and over to the side, pointing it toward the floor in front of you. Repeat on both sides for 30 seconds each time, then switch legs and repeat again. This stretch is good for improving flexibility and increasing circulation in the hips.

Raise one arm overhead and reach toward the opposite side of the room.

This stretch is great for improving your flexibility, especially if you have a tight chest or shoulders. It also works to open up your lungs and improve breathing capacity by increasing lung capacity.

Hold the stretch for 30 seconds on each side.

- Lie on your back with both legs straight and arms stretched out to the sides, palms facing up.

- Bring one knee up toward your chest and grasp it with both hands; then pull it toward you until you feel a gentle stretch in your hamstrings (the muscles behind your thighs).

- Hold this position for 30 seconds while breathing deeply through your nose, then switch sides and repeat with the other leg.

Cat and Cow

Cat and Cow is a simple, yet effective exercise that stretches the spine and abdomen. It also strengthens the abdominal muscles and improves posture.

Begin by kneeling on all fours with your hands directly under your shoulders, knees under hips, and forehead touching the floor or mat. Inhale as you slowly arch back like an angry cat stretching its back--this is cow pose! Then exhale as you round forward like a contented cow lying down in its field--this is cat pose! Repeat this movement several times until it becomes easy for you to do so without thinking about it too much (about 10 reps).

Cat Stretch

The cat stretch is a great way to get your spine moving. This exercise is also known as the "cat-cow" because it resembles the movement of a cat stretching, then relaxing.

Start on all fours with your hands directly under your shoulders and knees below your hips. Inhale, lifting your head and tailbone up toward the ceiling while dropping your belly down toward the floor. Exhale as you round over like a cat curling into itself before relaxing back into an arch position again. Repeat this motion several times until you feel loose in every joint!

Downward Dog

Downward Dog is a great way to stretch your body and wake up your muscles. It's also a good way to do this exercise when you don't have a lot of time because it only takes about one minute.

- Stand with your feet hip-width apart, knees bent and hands on the floor in front of you (fingers pointing forward).
- Inhale as you lift up into an inverted "V" position with arms straight and heels lifted off the floor. Keep abs engaged throughout the entire movement, stretching through heels if possible.

Half Moon Pose

Half Moon Pose: This is a great stretch for your legs and back.

In this pose, you'll want to make sure that the front leg is bent at 90 degrees, with the knee directly over the ankle and foot turned out slightly so that it's parallel with the outer edge of your mat. Your back leg should be straight but not locked out; feel free to bend it slightly if needed in order to keep both hips square or even gently twist them open toward each other as much as feels comfortable for you!

From here, bring both hands up onto either side of your head (or hold onto a strap if necessary) while keeping shoulders down away from ears; then lean forward into an inverted V shape by engaging those glutes! Hold for 5-10 breaths before switching sides.

Runner's Lunge

Stand straight with your feet together, knees slightly bent and arms outstretched in front of you. Bend both knees as if about to sit down on an imaginary chair behind you, keeping the weight on the balls of both feet. Lower yourself until both knees are at least 90 degrees from straight; if that's too much or doesn't feel comfortable, stop when they're bent as much as they can comfortably go without causing pain in either leg (about 45 degrees). Hold this position for 30 seconds before returning back up into a standing position. Repeat three times per day for best results!

Warrior 1

Warrior 1 is a great yoga pose that stretches your legs and hips. It also strengthens the arms and shoulders, which can help you feel more energized throughout the day. Here's how to do it:

- Stand with feet hip-width apart, knees slightly bent and arms at sides.

- Turn right foot 90 degrees out from body (toes pointing away from midline). Shift weight onto left leg as you bend right knee slightly; place top of right foot on floor about 3 inches behind left heel for support if needed. Press palms together in front of chest with fingers interlaced as shown above; keep chin parallel with floor throughout exercise--do not look up!

Warrior 2

Warrior 2 is a basic pose that's great for stretching your legs and opening up your hips. It also helps to strengthen the muscles in the back of your legs. Start by standing with your feet about hip-width apart, then bend both knees and bring them into a deep lunge position with one leg bent forward (like you're getting ready to jump) and the other bent behind you. Place both hands on the floor in front of you or hold them together at chest height if they are too tight to reach down. Lift up through the top of both thighs as well as through each foot as they point straight ahead while keeping both knees bent deeply throughout this exercise so that they don't lock out during any part of it

Morning stretching is an easy way to wake up your body in the morning.

This can help you feel better throughout the day and prevent injuries from occurring.

Stretching before bedtime is also beneficial, as it allows you to relax and fall asleep easier.

Chest stretches.

To do this stretch, stand with your back to a wall. Place one hand on the wall for support and raise your arms over your head until they are straight up. Bend forward at the waist until you feel a stretch in your chest muscles. Hold for 15 seconds then return to an upright position before repeating two more times.

Upward arm stretch

This is a great exercise to loosen up your shoulders and upper back. Stand with your feet hip-width apart and slowly raise both arms up overhead. Breathe in as you lift, hold for a few seconds, then breathe out as you lower back down. Repeat 10 times.

Backwards arm stretch

This is a great stretch for your shoulders, arms and back.

- Stand with feet shoulder-width apart.

- Bend over at the waist while keeping your back straight and head up, until you feel a gentle pull in your lower back area. Hold this position for 20 seconds.

- Now slowly raise one arm overhead as far as it will go without bending at the waist or letting your body sag forward. Hold this position for 15 seconds. Repeat with another arm.

Shoulder blade squeeze

This is a great stretch for your chest and shoulders. Stand with feet hip-width apart, then raise both arms above your head until they're parallel to the floor. With elbows bent and palms facing each other, slowly pull down on one side of your body until you feel comfortable tension in your chest muscles (don't push too hard). Hold this position for 30 seconds before switching sides.

These exercises will help you stretch out your muscles.

If you're a morning person and want to wake up your body with some stretching, these exercises will help you stretch out your muscles.

- The first exercise is called "Hands on Shoulders". Stand straight with feet apart and then place both hands on top of each shoulder. Inhale deeply as you raise one leg off the ground, extending it forward as far as possible without bending at the knee or waist until it reaches parallel with floor. Hold for 5 seconds then bring down slowly while exhaling deeply from lungs.

Set your alarm for 10 minutes earlier than you normally do.

When it goes off, get out of bed and stretch as much as possible in your room or even outside if it's warm enough.

Stretch and roll your neck, shoulders and arms.

- Stretch and roll your neck, shoulders and arms.

- Sit up straight with your feet flat on the floor. Gently stretch one arm overhead, reaching to the left side with your right hand and vice versa. Hold for 5 seconds and repeat 10 times in each direction.

- Next, gently rotate both shoulders in small circles while keeping your arms relaxed by your sides (10 times). Then lift them up slightly off of the chair seat so they form a 90-degree angle with their body; rotate back down again slowly until they are fully extended (10 times).

Do some gentle stretches for your toes, ankles and calves.

- Stand with your feet hip-width apart and your arms by your sides.

- Bend one knee to a 90-degree angle, keeping the other leg straight.

- Bring both hands together in front of you as if they were praying; then bend at the waist as far as you can go without straining or feeling pain in either ankle or knee joints. Hold this position for 30 seconds before repeating on other side.

Take a few deep breaths to wake up properly.

- Take a few deep breaths. Try to breathe in through the nose and out through the mouth, taking care to exhale fully. This will help you wake up properly, as well as calm yourself down if you're feeling anxious or stressed out.

- Stretch for about five minutes before getting out of bed (or whenever else you can fit it into your morning routine). Stretching helps loosen up tight muscles that may have been strained during sleep, which makes them more flexible as well as less prone to injury later on in the day when they're under stress again--and who doesn't want that?

It's easier to wake up when you do these stretches in the morning.

You're probably used to waking up and stretching in the morning, but you may not be doing it as effectively. You know that when you stretch out your muscles, they're more flexible and less likely to become injured. But did you know that stretching in the morning can help wake up your body? It is true!

When we sleep at night our bodies go through a cycle of muscle relaxation and tension as we move through REM (rapid eye movement) sleep stages. This cycle happens several times throughout the night, which means that by morning most people have spent quite a bit of time with their muscles relaxed--which makes them stiffer than they were when they went to bed! That's where stretching comes in: when we stretch our muscles right after waking up (or even before going back to sleep), we help break up this tension cycle so that when we get up again later on in the day our bodies feel more refreshed than if they'd been left alone all night long without any attention paid toward keeping them flexible

Seated Side Stretch

- Sit on the floor, with one leg extended and the other bent so that your heel is touching your butt.

- Lean to the side, reaching for your toes with both hands. You can also keep one hand in front of you and one behind if it is easier to balance yourself that way.

- Hold this stretch for 30 seconds or more, then switch sides and repeat!

Reach Overhead Stretch

- Stand with feet shoulder-width apart and arms at your sides.

- Raise your right arm above your head, bringing it down behind you until you feel a stretch in the front of that side of your body (the chest and shoulder muscles). Hold for 15 seconds.

- Repeat with left arm.

Standing Quad Stretch

Stand with your feet shoulder-width apart and knees slightly bent. Lift one foot off the ground, keeping it straight. Lean forward at the waist until you feel a stretch in the front of your thigh. Hold for 20 seconds and repeat with other leg.

Downward-Facing Dog Pose

The downward dog is a very common exercise and can be done anywhere. It stretches your legs, back and arms while strengthening them at the same time. This pose helps to strengthen your core muscles as well. You should try doing this pose for at least five minutes or until it becomes easy for you to hold the pose comfortably

Try these stretches when you wake up.

When you wake up, it's normal to feel stiff and sore. But stretching can help you feel better and even prevent injuries. Try these stretches when you wake up:

- Neck: Turn your head from side to side for one minute, then tilt your chin down toward your chest for one minute. Repeat this twice more, alternating directions each time (right, left; left, right).

- Shoulders: Roll them forward three times; roll them backward three times; then lift both arms above your head with palms facing each other and stretch them straight out (like an airplane flying), keeping them parallel with the floor for 30 seconds before lowering them again so that they're shoulder height on either side of your body as if holding onto a pole in front of you--hold this position for another 30 seconds before bringing both arms back down by your sides again.

Stretch your shoulders and neck

- Stretch your shoulders. Stand up straight, with your arms at your sides. Raise both hands above your head and interlock them, palms facing forward. Bend forward from the waist as far as you can without straining or feeling pain in any muscles. Hold this position for five seconds, then slowly return to a standing position.

- Stretch your neck. Sit up straight in a chair with both feet flat on the floor, knees bent at 90 degrees (or more). With one hand on either side of your head, gently pull back on each earlobe until you feel a slight stretch in the front of your neck; hold this position for 10 seconds before releasing it and repeating three times per side.

Stretch your chest and back

Stretching your chest and back is a great way to wake up. It stretches the muscles that are used when you're sitting at a desk all day, helping them relax and unwind.

To stretch your chest, stand with feet hip-width apart and raise both arms straight overhead with palms facing down toward the floor. Pressing gently into your heels, lift through the top of your head as you bend forward from the waist to touch either shin or toes (or as close as possible). Hold for 30 seconds then release slowly back into standing position before repeating on other side.

Focus on your arms, hands and fingers

Your arms, hands and fingers can be a great place to start.

- Stretch your arms out wide. Make a big "O" shape with your hands, then bring them back together in front of you with palms facing upward. Breathe deeply into this stretch for 30 seconds before repeating it on the other side of your body.

- Hold each hand out straight in front of you, then gently bend at the wrist so that they're pointing down toward the floor (like they're reaching for something). Slowly lower them until they reach their lowest point without pain or discomfort--you should feel this stretch along each forearm from elbow to wrist--

and hold it there for 30 seconds before raising back up again slowly; repeat three times total per side if possible!

Stretch your legs.

Stand with your feet hip-width apart and raise one arm over your head, stretching it toward the floor. With the other hand, grab onto a chair or table for balance. Lift up onto the toes of one foot and hold this pose for 10 seconds before switching to the other side. Repeat five times on each leg for a total of 10 reps per stretch (5x).

Morning stretching can help you feel more energized and relaxed.

Stretching in the morning can help you feel more energized and relaxed. It is a great way to start your day off on the right foot, especially if you're prone to feeling stiff or tense in the morning from sleeping in an awkward position (or even just because of aging). Here are some simple stretches that will loosen up tight muscles:

- Chest stretches: Stand with feet shoulder-width apart and place hands on hips. Then bend forward at waist until chest touches thighs or knees--whatever feels comfortable for you! Breathe deeply for 30 seconds as you hold this position before slowly returning upright again
- Side stretch: Stand with feet shoulder-width apart and arms extended straight out from sides at shoulder height; inhale as you raise one arm above head while bending over slightly towards same side (you should feel stretching in inner thigh), then exhale as return arm back down while keeping another arm elevated.

Stretch It Out

Stretching is an important part of your warm-up routine. Stretching helps to improve flexibility, range of motion and can even reduce soreness after a workout.

There are several unusual ways to stretch: static, dynamic and PNF (proprioceptive neuromuscular facilitation). Dynamic stretches involve moving through a range of motion with continuous movement such as bending at the waist while reaching towards your toes or swinging one arm overhead while keeping the other arm straight out in front at shoulder height for 30 seconds before switching sides. Static stretches are held for 10-30 seconds per muscle group; this requires you to relax into each stretch until you feel tension release throughout your body followed by holding the position without bouncing or swaying (this is where you'll find that "tension relief" feeling). Lastly PNF involves holding a passive stretch then contracting against resistance provided by an external force such as gravity or another person's hands until tension releases again before relaxing back into place

Roll It Up

- Sit on the floor with knees bent and feet flat on the floor.
- Place one hand behind your back, allowing it to rest against the lower back for support. Place other hand on top of thigh or knee.
- Roll forward until spine is straight and shoulders are relaxed (do not overextend).

Get Down on All Fours

- Stretch your back and hamstrings by getting down on all fours and reaching for your toes. This can also be done with a slight knee bend, allowing you to stretch deeper into the muscles in the backs of your legs.

The Seated Twist

The seated twist is a gentle stretch that can be done at your desk. Sit up straight, then take one arm behind your back and grab onto the opposite elbow with that hand. Then, gently pull the elbow toward the opposite knee until you feel a stretch in your lower back and hip muscles.

This exercise is also known as "twisting" because it involves twisting from side to side while sitting down on a chair or bench (or even standing up). In order to do this, move properly and safely, make sure that there aren't any objects nearby that could cause injury if hit accidentally by one of your limbs during rotation!

Hamstring Stretch with a Wall

Stretching your hamstrings can be a challenge. The muscles in the back of your legs are very tight, and they are prone to cramps if you don't stretch them regularly.

To do this stretch, stand facing a wall with one leg extended behind you and the other foot flat on the floor (a). Slowly bend at the knee of your extended leg until you feel a gentle pull on that side of your body (b). Hold for 30 seconds before switching sides.

Lunge Pose and Crescent Moon Pose

This is a great stretch for your hamstrings, calves and hips. It's also a good way to warm up before you start your day.

Stretching can help prevent injury.

When you're stretching, you want to make sure that your muscles are stretched gently and slowly. It's also important to breathe normally while stretching--don't hold your breath!

If a muscle feels tight or painful, stop immediately and don't stretch it further. If the discomfort persists after several minutes of rest, contact a medical professional for advice on how best to proceed with your exercise routine.

Hip Flexor Stretch

- Stand with your feet hip-width apart, knees slightly bent, and arms relaxed at your sides.
- Raise one leg off the floor and bend it so that the sole of your foot is pointing toward the ceiling.
- Hold this position for 30 seconds or longer before switching legs and repeating on other side.

Quadriceps Stretch

To stretch your quadriceps, sit down with one leg straight in front of you and the other bent at the knee at 90 degrees. Place one hand on top of the straight leg and use it to gently pull that knee toward the chest, keeping both hips facing forward. Hold for 15 seconds, then switch sides and repeat three times per side.

If this exercise is too difficult for you, try sitting on a chair instead of standing up and bending over--it's easier to hold onto something when you're seated!

Hamstring Stretch

- Stand with your feet shoulder-width apart.
- Bend your left leg and bring it behind you, so that the heel of your foot is on the ground.
- Bend forward at the hips, reaching for your toes with both hands if possible. If not, then just bring them as close as you can get them! Keep breathing deeply and slowly throughout this exercise.

Chest Stretch

This is a great stretch to do in the morning before you start your day. It is also good if you are feeling stiff or sore from exercising, working out or spending time at work.

To do this stretch, stand up straight with feet shoulder width apart and arms by your side. Inhale as you raise both arms above your head until they are parallel to the floor then exhale as you turn them outward so that each hand is facing away from each other at about 45 degrees (looks like an "X"). Hold for 15 seconds then repeat 3 times on each side

Shoulder Blade Stretch

One of the best ways to stretch your shoulders is to lie on your back with both arms straight out in front of you and palms facing down. Lift one arm up so that it's at least parallel to the floor, keeping the other arm on the ground. Hold this position for about 15 seconds before lowering your arm and repeating with the other side.

The Shoulder Blade Stretch

This is another great stretch for opening tight shoulders. Start by standing with feet hip-width apart and arms by your sides; then lean forward from your hips until there's a slight bend in both knees (but don't lock them), keeping chest lifted and core engaged throughout this movement! Hold this position for 15 seconds before switching sides.

Wrist and Forearm Stretch

To do this stretch, stand with your feet shoulder-width apart and hold a light weight in each hand. Raise the weights over your head and stretch the arms back as far as possible. Then slowly lower them down to the sides of your body, keeping them straight at all times. Repeat five times on each side for best results!

Chapter 4 – Evening Stretching Exercises

Stretching is an important part of fitness and health. It helps improve flexibility, maintain muscle tone, and reduce stress. Stretching before bed can help you sleep better, too! The following exercises are great for stretching out your muscles after a long day at work or school:

Begin with warm-up stretches.

- Warm up with some gentle stretches. Before you begin your workout, it is important to warm up your muscles. This will help prevent injury and allow you to get the most out of your exercise routine.
- Stretch while standing tall with feet hip-width apart, arms at sides (or on hips). Bend forward from the hips until you feel a stretch in the front of the thighs; hold for 10 seconds and then return to starting position. Repeat five times for each leg.

Stand up and back bends.

Stand up and back bends are a great way to stretch your muscles after sitting for long periods of time. If you have trouble doing this on your own, ask a friend or family member for help.

If you're not sure how to do a standing bend, here are some tips:

- Stand with feet shoulder-width apart.
- Bend forward at the waist until your hands touch the floor in front of you (or as close as possible). Hold this position for 10 seconds before slowly returning to standing upright again.

Arm stretches.

Stretch your arms out in front of you, then raise them above your head. Stretch one arm up and over, then the other. Repeat this stretch several times on each side before moving on to the next one.

Stretching exercises for legs:

Hamstring stretches.

- Lie on your back and bend one leg at the knee so that it's resting flat on the floor.

- Take hold of the other leg, and pull it toward you until you feel a stretch in your hamstring muscles (the muscle group behind your thighs). Keep breathing deeply as you hold this position for 15 seconds or more before slowly releasing and repeating with the second leg

Calf stretches.

This exercise is great for stretching the muscles in your lower legs. It can help improve flexibility and even reduce pain in your calves. To perform this stretch, stand upright with feet shoulder width apart on a flat surface (e.g., floor). Bend one knee up toward your chest while keeping both heels on the ground. Try to keep both knees straight throughout this exercise as much as possible; if necessary bend them slightly for comfort but do not round over at any point during this stretch! Hold this position for 30 seconds before switching legs and repeating.

Back stretches.

- Supine back stretch - Lie on your back with legs straight and arms extended forward at shoulder level. Bend one knee and place the foot on the floor, then pull it in toward your buttocks. Repeat with other leg.
- Twisting supine back stretch - Lie on your back with knees bent and feet flat on floor. Cross arms over chest or behind head so that they form an X shape across your body at about ear level, then turn to one side while keeping them in place throughout the movement (as if doing a sit-up). Repeat on other side of body by turning toward opposite direction of first twist; repeat once more for three total twists per set

Stretching is a great way to relax and prepare for sleep.

You can do these stretches at night before bed to help you relax and prepare for sleep.

Neck Stretch

This stretch is great for opening up your chest, shoulders and upper back. It also helps to improve posture by stretching the muscles in the front of your neck and shoulders. To do this stretch:

- Stand with feet shoulder-width apart (or wider) and knees slightly bent.
- Bend forward from the hips, keeping back as straight as possible without rounding it or arching it excessively; keep arms relaxed at sides with palms facing down toward floor; hold for 30 seconds to 1 minute before switching sides

Shoulder Stretch

The shoulder stretch is a great way to get your shoulders and upper back muscles loose.

- Place your arms behind you, palms facing out.
- Lift up one hand until it reaches the same height as your opposite knee. Hold this position for 30 seconds or more before switching sides and repeating with the other arm.

Chest Stretch

This is a great stretch to do before you go to bed, or as part of your morning routine. It helps open up the chest and shoulders, which can get tight from sitting at a desk all day.

Begin by standing with your feet together. Then, extend one arm straight out in front of you at shoulder height, palm facing down towards the floor. Reach up with the other hand and grab hold of it (or place it on top if that's more comfortable). Gently pull down on both arms until they're straight out in front again--but don't force anything here! You should feel some light tension in your chest muscles as they stretch outwards from their usual position against gravity; keep working until this becomes uncomfortable enough for release but not painful or dangerous-feeling in any way whatsoever!

This stretch is excellent for relieving tension in the lower back and improving posture. It can be done while sitting at your desk or standing up, depending on how much time you have available.

- Sit tall with legs crossed, hands resting on thighs (or knees if they don't reach).
- Inhale deeply through the nose and exhale slowly through pursed lips as you gently tilt your head toward one shoulder, then repeat with the other side.

Abdominal Stretch

To stretch your abdomen, lie on the floor and put your hands under your lower back. Lift your head and shoulders off the ground while keeping them in line with your hips. Breathe deeply for five to 10 seconds before relaxing back down onto the floor.

Repeat this exercise three times per day, holding each stretch for about 30 seconds at a time.

Hamstring Stretch

The hamstring stretch is a great way to relax and recover from the day. It can also help you get a good night's sleep, so try it before bedtime if you struggle with insomnia.

To do this stretch:

- Stand with your feet hip-width apart and arms at your sides, hands on hips or clasped behind your back (A).
- Lift one foot off the floor; bend both knees slightly as you reach toward that foot with both hands (B).
- Hold for 30 seconds before switching legs and repeating on other side (C).

These exercises can help you relax after a long day and stretch out your muscles.

Now that you know the benefits of stretching, here are some exercises that will help you relax after a long day and stretch out your muscles.

- The Cobra Pose: Lie on your stomach with arms stretched out in front of you. Lift up one arm and hold it there for five seconds, then lower it back down again before repeating with another arm. Do this 10 times (or more if comfortable).
- The Seated Twist: Sit with legs crossed in front of each other, hands resting on knees or thighs if possible--you want to keep them as straight as possible during this exercise! Now twist from side-to-side until feeling a good stretch in your back muscles; hold each position for 5 seconds before moving on to another one until done with all four directions around 360 degrees total (clockwise from North).

Seated twist

This is a great stretch for the obliques (the muscles on your side), as well as your lower back and hamstrings. Sit up straight with your legs extended in front of you, feet together or apart. Then place one hand behind you on the floor and reach the other arm across to grab it by its wrist, pulling until there's tension in your lower back-- but don't force anything! Hold this position for 30 seconds before switching sides

Child's pose

Child's pose is a relaxing stretch that can be done at any time of day. It can also be used to relieve stress and tension in the body.

- Kneel on the floor with your knees under your hips and your feet flat on the floor, about 2-3 feet apart from each other.

- Fold forward over your legs, placing your forehead on the mat or floor if possible. If this is too difficult for you, rest on folded arms instead.

Shoulder rolls

- Shoulder rolls: This is a great way to stretch your shoulders and upper back. You'll feel the tension release as you roll forward, then backward, then side to side.

- Neck stretch: In this exercise, you'll gently pull your chin toward one shoulder and hold for several seconds before switching sides.

- difficult or uncomfortable then place them on either side of one foot instead.

Downward-facing dog

Downward-facing dog is a great stretching exercise. It can be done in any room, and you don't need any equipment to do it.

To do downward-facing dog:

- Stand with your feet hip-width apart and hands on the floor in front of you, fingers pointing forward or slightly out to the sides.

- Raise up onto the balls of your feet and tuck in your tailbone as much as possible, so that there's an inverted V shape between your lower back and thighs (this isn't possible if you have tight hamstrings). Your body should form an upside down "V" shape from head to heels with no gap between them; keep those shoulders relaxed away from the ears!

Chair pose

Chair pose is a great way to open up your chest and shoulders.

- Stand with feet hip-width apart, knees slightly bent.

- Reach arms overhead, interlace fingers, and press palms together.

- Lift the chest slightly while keeping the spine long (you should be able to see between your hands). Hold for 5-10 breaths before releasing back into downward dog or child's pose if desired.

Lunge stretch with both arms overhead

Lunge Stretch with Both Arms Overhead

- Stand with your feet about hip-width apart, then step your right leg back into a lunge. Make sure that the front knee does not go past your toes and keep it bent at a 90-degree angle.

- Bring both arms overhead, reaching up toward the sky while keeping your chest open and shoulders relaxed. Stay in this position for 30 seconds before returning to starting position and repeating on the other side of your body.

Chest opener with hands on the floor outside the front foot.

The chest opener with hands on the floor outside the front foot is a great way to stretch your chest and shoulders.

- Sit on your mat with your legs extended in front of you.

- Bend both knees so that both feet are flat on the floor and bring them towards each other until they're touching. If this isn't possible, use props like blocks or cushions under each ankle if needed.

- Fold forward over one leg at a time until both forearms come into contact with the floor beneath them (or as close as possible).

Stretch your shoulders and biceps.

- Stand with your legs shoulder-width apart, arms at your sides.

- Raise both arms straight out to the sides until they're parallel to the floor (or as far as you can go without straining).

- Hold this position for 30 seconds or longer if comfortable--it's okay if it feels like too much!

Stretch your calves and shins.

- Stretch your calves and shins.

- Stand with your feet hip-width apart and toes facing forward.

- Bend one leg, placing the heel of that foot on the ground behind you as far as it is comfortable. Keep both knees straight and lean forward from the hips until you feel a stretch in your calf muscles. Hold for 30 seconds or more; repeat with other leg.

Quadriceps stretch.

Stretch your quadriceps by lying on your back with one leg bent, the other straight and both feet flat on the floor. Pull your heel towards your buttocks as far as possible without straining. Hold for 30 seconds and repeat with other leg.

Chest and shoulder stretch

- Stand with your feet hip-width apart.

- Bend your right arm and place it behind your back, palm facing up.

- Bend at the waist and lean over, reaching toward the floor with both hands. Hold for 15 seconds while breathing deeply through your nose or mouth (whichever is more comfortable). Repeat on opposite side.

Neck stretches.

- Neck stretches.

- Sitting up straight, slowly tilt your head to the right. Hold for 5 seconds and then repeat with the left side of your neck. Do this 3 times on each side of your neck.

Calf and ankle stretch.

Stretch your calves and ankles.

To stretch your calves, stand on a step or chair with your feet shoulder-width apart and toes pointing forward. Lift up onto the balls of your feet, hold for 10 seconds, then lower back down slowly. Do this 10 times per foot (20 total). To stretch your Achilles tendon and plantar fascia in the bottom of each foot, place one heel on a step or box with both knees bent and lean into it until you feel a gentle pull--but do not push too hard! Hold this position for 15-30 seconds before switching sides and doing another 15-30 seconds on each side again (60 seconds total).

Neck Rolls

To stretch the neck, roll your head slowly to one side. Hold for 5 seconds, then roll to the other side and hold for 5 seconds. Repeat this exercise 10 times in each direction.

Inner thighs: Stand with your feet hip-width apart and knees slightly bent. Clasp your hands behind you, and bring them to rest on the top of your buttocks. Gently press into the muscles between each buttock, lifting through the spine as you do so. Hold for 10 seconds then release slowly back down into a squatting position (see below). Repeat three times for each leg.

Outer thighs: The outer thigh muscles are often neglected during stretching because they are difficult to access without assistance from someone else or by using props such as a wall or chair--but this doesn't mean they should be neglected! To stretch these muscles independently of others nearby, lie face up with one leg bent at about 90 degrees and resting on top of its opposite number; keep both feet flat on the floor throughout this exercise so that only one set of joints moves at any given time (you'll feel some pressure in both sets). Bend forward toward knee while pressing gently against inner thigh muscle until stretch is felt in front portion where quadriceps meet hamstrings; hold stretch for 30 seconds before releasing slowly back down into starting position

Chapter 5 – Stretching the upper body

Stretching exercises improve flexibility and increase blood flow to your muscles.

Stretch the front of your chest.

To stretch your chest, stand upright and place one hand on your chest. With the other hand, pull down gently but firmly until you feel a stretch in your chest. Hold for 10 seconds, then release and switch sides.

Stretching the front of your body will help you breathe better and improve posture--so do it often!

Stretch your triceps and upper back.

It's important to stretch both the front and back of your arms, as well as their corresponding muscles. Stretch by reaching toward the ceiling with one arm, then pull that elbow across in front of you with the other hand. Hold for 10 seconds or until you feel a slight stretch in your triceps muscle (the muscle behind your upper arm). Then switch sides and repeat on each side three times each day.

Stretch the sides of your torso.

- Stretch the sides of your torso.

- Stand with feet hip-width apart, hands at your sides.

- Inhale as you lift arms overhead, keeping them straight (or bent slightly).

- Exhale as you lean over to one side, bringing that hand down to touch the ground behind you; then repeat on other side.

Stretch your shoulders and upper arms.

- Stretch your shoulders and upper arms.

- Sit on a chair or bench with your feet flat on the floor and knees bent at a 90-degree angle. Put one hand on each knee, then straighten the arm closest to you so it's perpendicular to the ground (your elbow should be pointing toward the ceiling). Now rotate that arm outward until you feel a stretch in your chest muscles; hold for 15 seconds before switching sides. Repeat two more times with each arm.

- Stretch your wrists by holding one arm out and the other in.

- Sit on a chair and hold one foot in front of you with both hands, then pull it backwards until you feel a stretch on your calf muscle (the back of your leg). Hold for 10 seconds, then switch legs.

Stretch your forearms by firmly grasping something with both hands, and hold for 30 seconds.

This stretch will help you to avoid injury during activities that require gripping strength, such as weightlifting or rock climbing.

Stretch your back with a towel or rope tied to something stable, then wrap it around you and pull gently.

This stretch is great for opening up your shoulders and upper back. You can do it standing or seated on the floor.

Hold one arm behind you as far as possible, then pull it forward, stretching the muscles on that side of your body. Repeat with another arm.

Roll your head from side to side for better neck mobility.

Stretching the neck can be a challenge, but it's important to keep your spine flexible and mobile. If you don't stretch regularly, a stiff neck can lead to other problems like headaches and back pain. To improve flexibility in this area of the body:

- Sit or stand with good posture and place one hand on either side of your head (see photo).
- Slowly roll your head toward one shoulder, then return it to center before rolling in the opposite direction. Repeat five times on each side if possible; otherwise, three times is enough if that feels comfortable for you!
- Stretching can improve flexibility and circulation in your upper body, reducing the chance of injury when exercising.
- Stretching also helps to relax tense muscles, which can reduce stress and make you feel more at ease.

The neck is a very flexible part of the body, but it can be very vulnerable. The muscles that support your head and neck are not as strong as those in other parts of your body. If you hold a heavy object on one side of your body for a long time, it's easy to strain or even tear these muscles.

You should stretch out before doing any exercise that involves raising or lowering your arms over head (such as weight lifting). This will loosen up the tightness in these areas so that there isn't too much pressure on them during exercise--and afterward as well!

Correct posture is important for both your mental and physical health.

When you slouch, it's like telling your body that it's okay to be unbalanced. As a result, you'll feel more fatigued and less energized throughout the day.

The best way to improve posture is by making small changes like sitting up straight at work or standing tall when talking to someone on the phone or in person. If these simple adjustments don't seem like enough of an improvement on their own, try doing some stretches every morning before getting out of bed--they'll help loosen up any tight muscles that may have developed over time due to poor posture!

Maintaining good posture can help prevent pain and injuries throughout the body.

Maintaining good posture can help prevent pain and injuries throughout the body. It's important to stretch regularly, but you also need to work on your posture. Stand up straight with your shoulders back, chest out and knees slightly bent. Make sure that you lift heavy items with both hands rather than bending over from the waist with one arm extended out in front of you (this puts too much strain on the lower back).

Many people are physically active every day, but their desk jobs or other sedentary activities can cause them to develop bad habits that negatively affect their bodies. When you sit in one place for long periods of time, your body tends to become stiff and tight. This is because the muscles in our backs, legs and arms don't get enough exercise when we're sitting down all day long. If you want to keep your muscles healthy while working at a desk job or spending hours at home on the couch watching TV after work, then it's important that you stretch regularly throughout the day (and not just right before bedtime).

Stretching exercises improve flexibility and increase blood flow to your muscles.

This can help reduce the risk of injury and allow you to perform at a higher-level during exercise or sports.

Stretching also helps improve posture, balance, coordination, strength and endurance.

The following stretches are designed to stretch out your upper body:

Stretching is the best way to warm up your muscles and prevent injury. If you're new to stretching, we recommend starting with some simple stretches like these:

- Chest Stretch - Stand straight with feet shoulder-width apart and place hands on top of head with elbows out to sides (like an airplane). Gently pull shoulders back as far as comfortable while inhaling deeply through nose and exhaling through mouth until fully relaxed into position; hold for 10 seconds before releasing slowly back into basic standing position again; repeat 5 times total per set (each time you repeat this exercise counts as one set). This can also be done sitting down by crossing one leg over another ankle then leaning forward from hips until tension builds around chest area; hold for 10 seconds before returning upright again; repeat 5 times total per set (each time you repeat this exercise counts as one set).

Chest stretches.

The chest stretch is an effortless way to open your chest and shoulders. It's also great for opening up the spine, which can help improve posture.

To do this stretch, stand with legs together and arms outstretched in front of you at shoulder height. Breathe in deeply through the nose and exhale through pursed lips as you drop both arms down until they are parallel with the floor (don't let them hang). Hold this position for 20 seconds before returning to upright posture; repeat 8 times total.

Neck stretch

You can stretch the neck by placing both hands on the back of your head. Gently pull your chin down toward your chest and hold for about 30 seconds. Repeat this stretch two or three times per day to relieve tension in the neck muscles.

Shoulder stretch

The shoulder stretch is a great way to loosen up the shoulders after a long day of typing or mouse clicking.

The steps are as follows:

- Stand tall with feet hip distance apart and hands on hips, inhale deeply through your nose, then exhale fully through pursed lips (as if whistling). Repeat this three times before proceeding to step two.

Overhead stretch

This stretch can be done anywhere, but it's best to do it on a hard floor. If you have a mat or towel, that's even better.

- Lie down with your stomach flat against the floor and arms straight out in front of you at shoulder height (or higher).
- Bend one knee and bring that foot toward the opposite elbow until a stretch is felt in both sides of your upper body. Hold for 30 seconds to 1 minute; repeat with another leg/arm combo if desired!

These stretches can help you keep your muscles flexible.

You can stretch your upper body muscles with these simple exercises.

- Chest stretches: Stand up straight and put your hands on the hips. Lift one arm over the head and lean forward slightly, stretching that side of the chest. Hold for 5 seconds, then switch sides and repeat 10 times for each side of your body.
- Shoulder shrugs: Stand up straight with feet shoulder-width apart and hold weights (or use no weight if you don't have any) in each hand at shoulder height with elbows bent 90 degrees out to the sides of your body and palms facing down toward floor; raise shoulders toward ears as high as possible without arching back or lifting heels off ground; lower slowly back down through range of motion until arms hang straight down from shoulders again

Do a few forward bends.

- Do a few forward bends.
- If you've been sitting at a desk all day, it's important to stretch out the muscles in your back and neck. Forward bends are great for this because they allow you to gently lengthen those muscles without putting any strain on them--a perfect combination of relaxation and flexibility!

Reach for the sky.

This exercise is a great way to stretch your arms, shoulders and upper back. It can also help improve posture by strengthening these muscles which will then allow you to stand up straight with ease!

- Stand with feet shoulder-width apart, arms relaxed at sides
- Lift both arms above head with palms facing forward (like an airplane). Hold for 30 seconds or more

Stretch your torso.

- Stretch your torso.
- Stand with feet hip-width apart, knees slightly bent and arms at sides.
- Inhale as you raise both arms above head, palms facing forward; exhale as you lower into a deep lunge on right leg (knees bent 90 degrees). Hold for 30 seconds; repeat on left side.

Stretch your obliques.

- Stretch your obliques. The sides of the abdomen are called "obliques," and they're often neglected when it comes to stretching. Stretching them will help improve your posture, so you can stand up straight and proud! Here is how:
- Lie on your back with knees bent and feet flat on the floor. Pull in both knees toward chest, keeping them close together as much as possible. Hold for 30 seconds; repeat three times in each position for best results!

Stretch your glutes and hamstrings.

This stretch is one of the best for stretching your glutes and hamstrings. It is a great way to warm up before you start running, or even just as an active recovery day. You can also use this stretch after a run or other type of exercise when your muscles are already warmed up from activity.

The key to this stretch is keeping both knees pointing straight ahead while keeping them on the floor. If you have trouble doing this at first, try placing one foot under the opposite knee so that both feet are flat on the ground (but not crossed). This will help keep both knees pointing forward while still allowing some bend in each joint--a good position for beginners!

Stretch your quads, hip flexors and calves.

Stretching your quads, hip flexors and calves will help you avoid injury by increasing flexibility and reducing muscle tightness.

Quadriceps stretch: Stand with one foot in front of the other and reach toward your toes with both hands. Hold for 20 seconds, then switch legs.

Hip flexor stretch: With one leg bent at a 90-degree angle in front of you, lift up on that heel as high as possible without bending forward or twisting (it should feel like you're trying to touch the ground). Hold for 20 seconds then switch legs.

Calf stretches: Stand facing a wall with both feet together; place one hand against it for balance; raise up onto tiptoes by pushing off with toes until feeling a slight tension in calf muscles--but don't lock knees! Hold position 10-15 seconds then lower down slowly until heels rest flat again before repeating once more if needed

Chapter 6 – Stretching the lower body

Stretching is an important part of any workout routine. If you're like me, though, you might not always get around to it. But if you're reading this chapter, then I'm guessing that means that you want to start stretching more regularly! This post will give you some ideas for stretches that are easy enough for anyone at any level of fitness or flexibility—and it'll explain why those stretches matter so much too.

Hip flexors stretch.

The hip flexor stretch is a simple exercise that can be performed in just about any gym or home. It stretches the muscles on the front of your hips, which are often tight due to sitting for long periods of time.

- Stand with your feet wider than shoulder-width apart and toes pointed slightly outwards.
- Place one hand on a wall or chair behind you for support if needed. Lift one leg up behind you as high as it will go without letting that knee drop down towards the floor (you should feel this in your quadriceps). Hold for 30 seconds then switch sides.

Calf stretches.

- To stretch the calves, stand on your toes with your heels off the ground. Keep a straight back and arms at your side.
- Hold that position for 15-20 seconds before slowly lowering down onto your heels and repeating 3 times.

Bodybuilder's-style splits

Bodybuilder's-style splits are the most common type of stretching routine. The idea behind them is to make your muscles more flexible by increasing their range of motion, which can help prevent injury and increase performance.

Stretching is important for everyone, but it's especially essential for people who exercise regularly--whether you're a runner or Cross Fitter, yoga fanatic or weightlifter. Regular stretching will help improve your flexibility and strengthen your muscles so they are less likely to be strained during exercise.

Hamstring stretches.

The hamstring is a large muscle in the back of your thigh that helps you bend and straighten your knee. When it's tight, it can cause lower back pain and make it difficult to walk normally. This stretch will help loosen up those hamstrings so they don't feel so tight all day long!

- Stand with one foot about two feet behind you and slightly bent forward at an angle (you can use a chair for support). Bring your other leg up towards your chest, keeping both knees straight but not locked out--you should feel a stretch in both legs now.
- Hold this position for one minute before switching sides.

Quadriceps stretch.

The quadriceps stretch is one of the most common and effective stretches for flexibility. It can be done by anyone, at any time, and it's easy to remember.

Begin by standing up straight with feet together. Lift one leg behind you until it is parallel with floor or higher (as high as possible). Keep your back straight and chest out throughout this exercise; do not bend forward! Hold this position for 30 seconds before switching legs.

Stretching is an important part of your workout.

Stretching is an important part of your workout. Stretching helps to reduce muscle soreness and allows you to build strength in your muscles without overworking them. Stretching also helps to improve flexibility, which can lead to more effective workouts and faster results.

- To stretch your lower body: Stand with feet hip-width apart, knees soft (not locked) and hands on hips; reach left leg back as far as possible without letting it drop; hold for 20 seconds while breathing deeply into the bottom of the lungs. Repeat with right leg.
- To stretch upper back: Reach arms overhead, interlace fingers behind head; gently pull shoulders down away from ears while arching spine slightly forward until there's a slight tugging sensation in chest muscles; hold for 20 seconds while breathing deeply into lungs through nose only (do not lift chest).

Stretch your calves.

- Stand with your feet hip-width apart and knees slightly bent. Lift one foot off the ground, then bend at the waist so that it touches the floor in front of you. Repeat with both legs 10 times per side, then do 5 repetitions of raising up onto tiptoes while keeping heels on floor (this will help stretch calves).

Stretch the front of your thigh.

Stretch the front of your thigh by standing with one leg in front and bending forward at the hip, keeping both knees straight. Place hands on floor in front of you for support if needed, then lift up onto toes and hold for 30 seconds before returning to starting position. Repeat three times on each side.

Stretch the back of your leg.

- Sit on the floor with one leg extended in front of you and the other bent at the knee.
- Keep your back straight and lean forward toward your extended leg until you feel a stretch through your hamstrings. You can place both hands on top of each other behind your thigh for support or rest them on top of each other in front of your knee for more assistance as needed.

Stretch your hips.

To stretch your hips, lie on the floor with your legs together. Bend one knee and place that foot flat on the floor. Place the other foot in front of you so that it's resting on its toes. Then lift both legs up until they form a 90-degree angle with each other at their intersection point (your pubic bone). Hold this position for 30 seconds before switching sides and repeating.

Seated Forward Bend

This is a simple stretch that can be done anywhere, anytime. It's perfect for people who don't have much flexibility in their hamstrings (the muscles on the back of your thighs) and calves. To do it:

Sit with legs straight out in front of you, toes facing up. Inhale deeply through your nose as you raise both arms above your head, stretching them toward the ceiling. As you exhale through pursed lips and rounded shoulders, bend forward from the hips until there is resistance in your hamstrings; keep knees slightly bent if necessary to avoid placing too much pressure on them. Hold this position for several breaths before returning upright again by extending arms down toward feet; repeat three times total for one set--or try holding each stretch for 30 seconds if possible!

Pigeon Pose

The pigeon pose is a great way to stretch the hips and thighs. It also strengthens the lower back and glutes, which can help improve posture.

Once you're in this pose, bring your hands behind your back and grab onto opposite elbows. Twisting from side to side will help open up the hips even more!

Warrior 3

Warrior 3 is a great pose to open up the hips and stretch the legs. It's also one of the easiest poses to do--as long as you don't fall over!

Step 1: Stand with your feet together, knees slightly bent and arms at your sides. Lift your left leg up so that it's parallel with the floor, then bend at the knee until it forms a 90-degree angle with your right leg (or as close as possible). Keep both heels planted on the ground throughout this pose; if necessary, place something under one or both heels for support.

Step 2: Place both hands on top of each other in front of your chest or heart center (this can vary based on body type). Inhale deeply through both nostrils while lifting up through all four corners of each foot; exhale completely out through pursed lips while relaxing all muscles in preparation for entering into Warrior 3 proper!

Half Moon Pose

Half Moon Pose is a great way to stretch your lower body and hips.

This pose can be done with either the right or left foot on top of the other, depending on which side of your body you need to stretch.

Tree Pose

The Tree Pose is a great way to stretch and strengthen your lower body. It also helps improve balance, flexibility and concentration.

To do this pose: Stand with feet together and hands on hips. Bend forward from the waist until you can grab hold of the big toes or ankles with each hand (if possible). Gently pull back on each foot until you feel a stretch in your quadriceps (thigh muscles). Keep knees slightly bent as you hold this position for 30 seconds to one minute

- Wide-legged forward fold
- One-legged squat with hands on a wall (or chair) for support

Hip Flexor Stretch

The hip flexor stretch is a great way to loosen up those tight muscles in your groin area. It's also a great exercise for runners, who often have tight hips because they spend so much time running on their toes. To do this stretch:

- Stand with feet shoulder-width apart and knees slightly bent.
- Lift one foot off the floor, keeping that knee bent at 90 degrees (not straight). You should feel some tension in your thigh muscles as you lift your leg higher than parallel with the floor--this is good! That means you're stretching out those hip flexors well!

Try these stretches to loosen up your lower body.

The lower body is made up of the muscles and joints that are located below your waist. This includes the hips, thighs, ankles and feet. These areas can become stiff from sitting at a desk all day or from not stretching after exercise. Stretching these muscles will help improve flexibility and help prevent injury when you're getting back into a fitness routine after taking some time off.

Here are some stretches to try:

- Hip flexor stretch (pictured above). Lie on your back with one leg straight and the other bent at 90 degrees while holding onto its ankle with both hands. Lift up your torso until it's aligned with both legs; hold for 30-60 seconds before switching sides. Hamstring stretch (pictured above). Start by sitting on floor with legs extended in front of you; cross right foot over left leg so toes touch floor; place hands behind neck or lower back for support as needed; press down through heels as far as comfortable without rolling pelvis forward (this avoids arching spine); hold 20 seconds or until discomfort subsides; repeat 3 times per side. Quadriceps stretch (pictured above). Sit on floor with knees bent 90 degrees so shins rest flat against surface behind them; place left hand behind head then reach forward toward right foot until slight pull is felt at bottom part of thigh muscle (don't force stretch); hold 15 seconds then switch sides

Inchworm

The inchworm is a great exercise for stretching the lower body and improving flexibility. It's also a good warm-up before running or other cardio exercise, as it helps loosen tight muscles in the hips and thighs.

To do this stretch: Stand with your feet together, knees slightly bent and arms at your sides. Slowly bend forward from the waist until you're in an upside-down V shape with only your hands touching the floor (or mat). Lift one foot off of the ground; keep both knees straight as you hold this position for 10 seconds before bringing it back down again. Repeat with opposite leg for 1 minute total time -- or until you feel like moving on!

Standing quad stretch

This exercise stretches the quadriceps and hamstrings, two muscle groups that can become tight and sore after running. To perform this stretch:

- Stand with one leg in front of the other, both feet facing forward.
- Bend your back leg so that it is at a 90-degree angle and place both hands on the knee of your bent leg for support (you may also want to place one hand on top of the other).
- Lean forward until you feel a stretch in your front thigh muscles; hold for 30 seconds or longer if possible

Lateral lunge

The lateral lunge is a great way to stretch the hip flexors and quadriceps. It's also a low-impact exercise that can be done with or without weights, making it an ideal warmup for more intense movements later in your workout.

To perform this move: Stand with feet together and arms at sides; step right foot out wide (about 4 feet), bending both knees until left thigh is parallel with floor. Keep torso upright and press down into right heel; return to start position, then repeat on opposite side (lunge).

Yoga is an amazing form of exercise that can help you improve your physical health, but it's also a great way to relax and unwind. The key thing about yoga is that it doesn't require any special equipment or clothing--you just need yourself! So, if you're looking for something new in your life, try taking up yoga classes at a local studio or gym.

Standing hip flexor stretch

Stand with your feet hip-width apart and bend forward at the waist. Rest your hands on a chair in front of you, or hold onto a wall or other sturdy object for support.

Hold this position for 30 seconds to 1 minute, breathing deeply throughout the stretch.

Standing quadriceps stretch

To stretch your quadriceps, stand with one leg in front of the other. If you're right-handed, place your left foot behind your right knee and grab hold of the back of that knee with both hands. If you're left-handed, do the opposite: place your right foot behind your left knee and grab hold of it with both hands.

Hold this position for 30 seconds while breathing deeply into any tight spots that feel like they need more attention (like where I'm holding my own leg here). Then switch sides and repeat!

Glute bridge

The glute bridge is a great exercise for stretching the lower body. It can help you improve flexibility, relieve tightness and prevent injuries.

- Lie on your back with knees bent and feet flat on the floor.
- Place hands under lower back for support if needed, but don't pull too hard or you may feel strain in the neck muscles instead of a stretch in your hips.
- Squeeze glutes (buttocks) together to lift hips into bridge position--you should feel tension between hamstrings and buttocks muscles working as you lift up off ground

Hip flexor-adductor stretch.

The hip flexor-adductor stretch is a great way to open up the hips and groin area. In this stretch, you'll be using your hands to pull one leg toward your chest while keeping the other leg straight on the floor in front of you. From there, gently lean forward until there's a slight stretch in the front of both legs (you may want to place an additional pillow or towel under your head). Hold this position for 30 seconds before switching sides!

There are a lot of stretches that can be done to work on tightness in your lower body.

- The quadriceps stretch is a great way to loosen up the muscles on the front of your thighs. Stand with one foot in front of the other and place both hands on top of the knee of your back leg. Bend forward at the waist until you feel a stretch in front of that thigh. Hold for 30 seconds, then switch sides and repeat twice more for each leg (three total). This exercise can also be done sitting down by crossing one leg over another and pulling gently toward yourself until it feels like a good stretch; hold for 30 seconds before switching legs and repeating two more times on each side (a total of three times per leg).

- Hip flexor stretches are effective at loosening up tight hip flexors--the band-like muscles between your pelvis bones that connect with large muscles at either end: iliopsoas muscle group at top; rectus femoris muscle group underneath--and help prevent injury when running or walking uphill especially if done regularly prior to activity such as walking around campus all day long while carrying books everywhere! To do these simple yet highly effective stretches simply sit down then lift one knee up slowly until there's tension felt alongside thigh where it meets pelvis bone area called pubic symphysis joint region which should feel like firm pressure but no pain whatsoever so don't force anything too far beyond this point otherwise risk damaging soft tissue structures within area which could lead serious problems later down line including arthritis type symptoms due repeated use over time despite precautions taken now!"

Split squat to lunge.

This exercise is a little bit more complicated than the previous two, but it is still pretty simple. The split squat to lunge combo will help you stretch the muscles in your lower body and improve flexibility. To begin, stand with feet shoulder-width apart and hold an 8–10-pound dumbbell in each hand (or use no weight at all).

Place one foot back about two feet behind you, then bend both knees until they are at 90 degrees or less. Make sure that your front knee does not extend past your toes as this can cause injury!

Now press through both heels while keeping them firmly planted on the ground until you are standing straight up again; repeat for 10 reps per leg before moving on to step three below!

Lunge with a twist

The lunge with a twist is a wonderful way to stretch the lower body.

To do it, take a wide stance and place your hands on your hips. Then, bend both knees and drop into a lunge until both thighs are parallel to the floor (or as far down as you can go without losing balance). To add an extra challenge, raise one leg off of the ground while keeping both feet flat on their respective sides. Hold this position for 10 seconds before switching legs and repeating on other side of body.

Elbow-to-knee lunge

To stretch your lower body, try an elbow-to-knee lunge.

Stand with feet hip-width apart and place one hand on a wall for balance. Step forward with one leg until the knee of that leg is bent at 90 degrees and the other leg is straight behind you. Lower yourself into a lunge until both knees are bent 90 degrees, then press through both heels to stand back up again. Repeat on opposite side (or alternate between sides).

This simple stretch can help improve blood flow throughout your legs and hips--which may reduce aches associated with sitting too long or standing all day at work!

Childs pose.

Child's pose is a great way to stretch the lower body. This pose can be done in several different ways, but the basic form is on your knees with your feet flat on the floor and your buttocks resting on your heels.

If you want to get more comfortable in child's pose, try placing a blanket under your knees or even folding up two blankets so that they support both sides of your body from head to foot.

These exercises will help you loosen up your lower body.

- The first exercise is a simple quad stretch. Stand with your feet hip-width apart and bend one knee up, keeping the other leg straight. Grab behind your thigh and pull it toward you until you feel a stretch in that quad muscle. Hold for 10-30 seconds then switch sides.

- The second exercise is an ankle mobilization exercise called "shoulder rolls." Kneel on all fours, then lift one knee off of the floor so that only one foot remains on the ground at a time (see photo). Next, roll both shoulders back as far as possible while keeping them level with each other and repeat this motion for about 20 reps per side.

Lunge stretches.

The lunge stretch is a great way to open up your hips and lower back. It's also a good way to prepare for more advanced stretches that require deeper flexibility in these areas, like the butterfly pose (a variation on the tree pose).

If you're new to yoga or stretching, start by sitting down with both legs straight out in front of you. Bend one knee so that it touches the ground directly under your hip joint--this will be your starting position for this stretch. From here, slowly lean forward until both arms are fully extended and parallel with the floor; hold this position until you feel some tension in your lower back or hamstrings (the muscles on either side of your rear leg), then release slowly back into place. Repeat three times before switching sides!

Quadriceps stretch.

- Place the right foot on a chair or bench and bend the left knee. Make sure that you're standing with your hips square to the floor and both feet pointing straight ahead (not turned out).

- Straighten the right leg as much as possible, keeping it in line with your body; hold this position for 30 seconds, then repeat with the other leg

Squatting lunge

This exercise will stretch your lower body.

To do this stretch, stand with feet hip-width apart and place one hand on a wall or chair for balance. Bend both knees until they are at 90 degrees and slowly lower yourself into a squatting position, keeping your back straight as you go down. Make sure to keep your weight in between both feet rather than placing all of it on one side (this will help prevent injury). Then rise back up by pushing through the heel of one foot while extending that leg behind you so that it forms an L shape with the other leg (make sure not to lock out either knee). When finished with this stretch, switch sides by moving away from where you started; repeat three times per side for optimal results!

Stretching the lower body is important to avoid injury.

There are a lot of ways to stretch your lower body, but the most important thing is to avoid injury. If you're not careful with how you stretch, it can be easy to overstretch and cause an injury. The best way to avoid this is by using proper technique when stretching and warming up before physical activity.

Stretching the lower body is especially important because it's easy for people who spend a lot of time sitting down (like office workers) or driving (like Uber drivers) to get tight muscles in their hips and thighs that are difficult for them to loosen up on their own.

Seated calf stretches.

This stretch is a great way to open up your calves and feet. It's also a good way to get ready for the seated toe touch exercise, which we'll get into later.

Sit on the floor with both legs straight out in front of you, toes pointed toward the ceiling. Place one hand on each knee for support, then lean forward until you feel a stretch in your calf muscles (this may take some time). Hold this position for about 30 seconds before switching sides and repeating with other leg extended out in front of you.

Bow-legged stance hip flexor stretches.

- Stand with your feet slightly wider than shoulder-width apart, toes pointing straight ahead.
- Inhale and lift your arms out to the sides at shoulder height.
- Exhale as you bend forward from the hips, keeping knees soft and chest lifted.
- Hold for 30 seconds on each leg; repeat 3 times (or rest in child's pose).

Standing toe touch stretch

Standing toe touch stretch

Stand with your feet hip-width apart and bend your knees slightly. Reach down and grab the toes of one foot with both hands, then pull them up toward your shin until you feel a stretch in the front of that leg. Repeat on both sides.

Calf stretches with resistance bands.

- Calf stretches with resistance bands.

- Step forward into a lunge and place one band around each ankle.

- Stand tall and keep your back leg straight, then step forward into a lunge with the other leg, keeping both knees bent at 90 degrees.

- Hold for 30 seconds, then repeat on the other side.

Hamstring and IT band stretches on a foam roller or ball

Hamstring and IT band stretches on a foam roller or ball.

The hamstrings are the large muscles in your lower legs that connect your upper leg to your lower back. If you have tight hamstrings, they can pull on the pelvis, which leads to discomfort in this area as well as lower back pain. To stretch them:

- Lie face down with one leg straight out behind you and the other bent at 90 degrees (or use two foam rollers if needed).

- Roll slowly up and down over the length of your hamstring muscle group until it feels stretched out enough for comfort--not too much! You might want to hold onto something for balance if possible so that both hands are free for rolling around safely on top of those hard plastic balls we call "foam rollers" or "medicine balls" here in America--and elsewhere around this great big world where such things exist...

Tight hip flexors can be a cause of back pain.

Tight hip flexors can be a cause of back pain. You may feel pain in your lower back when you lift your leg, or when you sit for long periods of time.

The best way to stretch these muscles is with a yoga pose called "the pigeon" or "eagle pose." This stretch should be done daily for five minutes at least three times per week to help alleviate tightness in the hips and lower back.

Tight hips can make it difficult to move properly and with power in your workouts.

When you're stretching your hips, it's important to keep in mind that there are many muscles in the area. The hip flexors, which run from the lower spine to the front of your hip bones, are often tight and can cause low back pain. Tight hamstrings (the muscles on the backs of your thighs) can also contribute to tightness in this region by pulling on those muscles when they're overstretched or underused.

To stretch all these areas effectively--and get more flexible overall--you'll need to take time out of every workout session for some dedicated stretching time.

It's also important to stretch after you exercise, because muscles are most pliable right after working out.

It's also important to stretch after you exercise, because muscles are most pliable right after working out. The best time to stretch is within 30 minutes of completing your workout (if you're doing it outside) or immediately before going to bed (if you've been working out at the gym).

Stretching shouldn't be painful, and should never hurt!

Stretching shouldn't be painful, and should never hurt. If you feel pain during your stretch, stop and consult a doctor.

Stretches that are too intense can actually cause harm to the muscles being stretched. This may lead to muscle tears or other injuries that could leave you sidelined for weeks or even months!

Chapter 7 - Stretching with equipment

Stretching exercises are important to help people feel better after exercising or working out!

Leg Press

The leg press is an excellent exercise for the quadriceps, hamstrings and gluteal muscles. It can also be used to help strengthen your core balance and stability. The machine allows you to add weight gradually as you become stronger, so it's perfect for those who are trying to build muscle mass or increase their overall strength.

The leg press works by placing your feet under the platform of the machine and leaning forward until your back touches against it before pressing upward with both feet simultaneously into a standing position again (or until you reach full extension).

Squats

This is a great exercise for your legs, back and core. It will help improve your flexibility and balance.

- Stand with feet hip-width apart, toes pointing forward or slightly outward.

- Bend at the knees until your thighs are parallel to the floor. Keep your back straight while bending down slowly; don't lean forward or backward as you squat down!

- Keep arms hanging loosely by sides during entire movement; do not let them swing up or down as you move into position (this can lead to injury).

- Return slowly until upright again; repeat 10 times total -- 5 times each leg

Chest Press

The chest press is a great exercise for strengthening the chest muscles. It works the pectoralis major and minor, as well as the anterior deltoid and triceps.

The machine shown in this picture is an example of a chest press machine, although many other types are available (such as free weights). Here's how you do it:

- Stand in front of your bench press station, facing away from it so that your back faces toward the mirror.

- Place one foot on each pedal, then grasp handles with both hands while keeping elbows slightly bent at all times throughout movement!

- Slowly lower weights until they're just below chin level before pressing them up again

Triceps Extension or Skull Crusher

This exercise can be performed using a cable machine or with dumbbells. It targets the triceps muscles at the back of your arm. To do this exercise, stand facing away from the weight stack and hold on to the bar with both hands. Start by bending your knees slightly and leaning forward at a 45-degree angle so that your upper body is parallel to floor while keeping knees bent slightly more than 90 degrees (keep them above your toes).

Stand up straight while extending arms up toward ceiling until they are fully extended with palms facing each other; then lower weights slowly down toward floor until elbows are nearly touching shoulders before repeating movement again.

Shoulder Press

The shoulder press is a great exercise for building your shoulders and upper back muscles. It also works your triceps, biceps and core muscles as well.

The equipment required for this exercise is a barbell with weights attached at each end. You can also use dumbbells if you prefer them over barbells but they will be heavier than using only one hand at a time instead of two like in this case so keep that in mind before starting out on any new workout routine where you might need help getting started if there isn't someone else around who knows what they're doing already (like if they've done these exercises before). If all goes well though then eventually we'll both be able to do all our own stretching exercises without needing anyone else around us anymore!

These are some of the best equipment assisted stretching exercises to help you stay flexible and fit.

- These are some of the best equipment assisted stretching exercises to help you stay flexible and fit.

- Stretching is an important part of any fitness routine, but it can be hard to find time in your busy schedule. Thankfully, there are many ways that you can incorporate stretching into your daily routine by using specialized equipment or machines. You don't have to go out and buy an expensive piece of machinery; many gyms offer these services as part of their membership packages or they may rent them out for a small fee (or even give them away). The following chapter lists some examples:

Why are use stretching equipment?

There are many reasons why you should use stretching equipment. For example, it's easier to keep track of your progress when you have a machine that measures how far and fast your muscles are moving. If you're trying to improve flexibility in one area or another, having a machine that tells you how much progress has been made makes it easier for people who aren't very flexible themselves because they can see what they need to work on next.

Another advantage is that these machines allow users who may not know how much force is too much or too little because they don't know their limits yet; this way, they won't hurt themselves while trying new things!

Stretching equipment can help you stretch deeper and move faster than stretching on your own.

You can get more out of your stretching by using equipment and machines. Stretching equipment will help you stretch deeper, move faster, and hold positions longer than if you were to do the same stretches on your own. Stretching with equipment also allows for greater flexibility in areas where it might be difficult or impossible to reach with just your own body alone.

- A strap is a long piece of fabric that's used to hold one part of the body while it works through an exercise routine or stretch session. Straps are usually made from leather, but there are some synthetic options available as well if you prefer those materials over animal products (and some people do). They're typically about 2 feet wide at their widest point so they fit comfortably around most people's bodies without being too tight or loose around any particular area where they might rub uncomfortably against tender skin surfaces like elbows/knees/wrists etc..

You can use machines to isolate muscles to make them work harder than you would otherwise, or to improve your range of motion. For example, if you're working out at home and don't have access to a personal trainer or stretching coach, working with resistance bands and dumbbells is an easy way for anyone with basic strength training knowledge (and some patience) to stretch safely at home.

One thing that should always be kept in mind when using any kind of equipment is that there are limits on how much weight should be lifted during each repetition; this varies based on the type of exercise being performed and whether it's intended as a warm-up or part of an intense workout routine.

Machines can be used in addition to free weight exercises to reduce stress on your joints and improve balance and control.

- Resistance machines are effective for strengthening the muscles of the arms, legs and back. They also help develop muscle endurance, which is important for maintaining good health. The main advantage of using resistance machines is that they allow you to perform multiple repetitions at a high intensity level without having to worry about stabilizing yourself against gravity (as with free weights). This allows you to work more efficiently than when using dumbbells or barbells alone.

- Weight-lifting machines offer safety benefits by limiting movement range so that users don't overextend themselves while exercising; this reduces injury risk compared with other forms of resistance training equipment such as barbells and dumbbells where there's no limit on how far movements may extend beyond their intended range of motion

Stretching equipment is useful for warming up before intense activity, and also for stretching after exercise.

- Before you start your workout, use a foam roller or massage ball to loosen up your muscles. This helps prevent injury by increasing blood flow and reducing soreness.

- After working out, stretch using the equipment shown above! These machines can help improve flexibility by stretching different parts of the body in one easy session (for example: hamstrings and calves).

Stretching machines are good for people who don't have much time or flexibility but still want a great workout

You can get a great workout with stretching machines. These machines are great because they allow you to stretch your muscles while using them, which is better than just sitting there and doing nothing! You'll feel energized and ready to go after using these machines.

Seated Chest Stretch

The seated chest stretch is a great way to loosen up your upper back, shoulders and arms.

- Sit on the floor with your legs bent in front of you and feet flat on the floor. Place one hand behind each knee for support and lean forward until you feel a gentle stretch in your chest area.

- Hold for 30 seconds then switch sides for another 30 seconds.

Chest Stretch on Incline Bench

- Lie face down on an incline bench, with your head resting on the top. Keep your arms straight by your sides and hold a light dumbbell in each hand (the weight should be heavy enough to challenge you).

- Lift the dumbbells straight up until they are level with the top of your chest, then lower them back down slowly without letting them touch the floor at any time during this exercise's range of motion (ROM). Repeat for 10-15 reps per set

Chest Stretch on Flat Bench

To stretch your chest, lie on a flat bench with your feet flat on the floor and you're back resting against the pad. Your arms should be hanging down by your sides with palms facing forward. Slowly raise both arms up toward the ceiling until they are parallel to it; hold for 30 seconds and then return to starting position. Repeat 10 times before switching sides and repeating exercise again for other side of body (right).

Seated Shoulder Stretch (External Rotators)

- Sit on the floor with your knees bent and feet flat.

- Grasp a towel in each hand and cross them over one another behind your back, so that they form an X shape.

- Bend forward at the waist until you feel a stretch in your shoulders and upper back muscles. Hold for 30 seconds to 1 minute before releasing slowly and repeating on other side.

Lying T-Spine Mobilization with Barbell Roll

This exercise is a great way to mobilize your thoracic spine. It can be done on a table or with the barbell in front of you, but I prefer it with the barbell because it's easier to control and allows me to feel where my range of motion is being limited.

Place your arms behind your head, then roll onto one side until you feel a stretch through the upper back. If this doesn't work for you, try rolling onto both sides at once by putting both hands behind your head and lifting up slightly off of each hip (like in cobra pose). Hold this position for 30 seconds before switching sides and repeating for 3-5 sets total per day

Side-Lying Clamshells with Resistance Band

Lie on your side and place the resistance band just above your ankles. Bend one knee and pull it up so that the foot is in front of you, then lift the other leg off of the floor. Repeat this motion for 10-15 repetitions on each side, alternating between sides as you go.

Supine Hip Extension

This exercise is a fantastic way to improve your hip extension. It also stretches the muscles of your lower back, hamstrings, and gluteal.

- Lie on your back with your legs straight and arms at your sides. Your feet should be about 12 inches apart from each other, with heels firmly planted on the floor.
- Lift knees off of the floor so that only toes are touching (or as close to this position as possible). Maintain this position for 10 seconds before lowering back down slowly into starting position again over 10 seconds' time.

Prone Iliopsoas and Quadriceps Stretch (1)

This stretch is great for the iliopsoas muscle, which runs from your hips to your lower back. You'll need a towel or piece of rope for this one.

- Place your right leg on top of your left knee so that they form an X shape.
- Wrap the towel around both ankles and gently pull them apart until you feel a stretch in your groin area and thigh muscles (the quadriceps). Hold for 30 seconds then switch sides.

Prone Iliopsoas and Quadriceps Stretch (2)

For this exercise, you'll need a bench or chair.

- Sit on the floor with both legs straight in front of you and feet together.
- Place one hand on each knee for support as you lift your hips up off the floor until they are in line with your torso.
- Hold for 15 to 20 seconds before lowering down again. Repeat three times per day, every other day or as directed by your doctor or physical therapist

Lift your right knee and pull it toward your chest.

Take a deep breath, and then exhort your body to relax.

Now, it's time to do some stretching!

Get on the floor and lie on your back with both legs extended in front of you. Make sure that the soles of both feet are touching each other, with knees bent at about 90 degrees. This is called "the child's pose" because it looks like an adult version of how babies sleep when they're lying down--you may have even seen this position in movies where someone is being murdered by an evil spirit (or just really angry parents).

If this feels too difficult for you right now, try sitting up against a wall instead; it will give more support than lying down does but still allow for some flexibility when moving around later on if needed during other activities such as eating breakfast or going outside without pants on--which isn't recommended unless absolutely necessary because pants help protect us from getting sunburned when outdoors during summertime temperatures above 100 degrees Fahrenheit which would result in death if exposed long enough without protection such as clothing made specifically designed specifically designed

Leg Extensions

This is a great exercise for building up your quads and hamstrings. It's also a good way to stretch out your hip flexors, which can become tight from sitting at a desk all day. The key is to keep your back straight as you lift yourself up on the machine, and make sure you don't swing or bounce as you lower yourself down again.

Seated Hamstring Curls

The seated hamstring curl is a great exercise for stretching your hamstrings. The seated position helps you to keep your back straight and avoid straining the lower back.

- Place one end of the resistance band under your feet. Stand on it with both feet together and hold onto both ends of the band in each hand at shoulder height (or higher). Keep your knees slightly bent, but don't lock them!

- Keeping your chest up, hips square and heels flat on floor throughout entire movement; slowly bend forward until you feel a stretch in hamstrings or glutes (you may need to adjust how far you reach down by moving closer/further away from anchor point). Hold for 2-3 seconds before returning upright again with control; repeat 8-10 times per set

Lying Leg Curls

This exercise works the hamstrings and lower back. It is performed by lying on your back with legs straight, feet flat on the floor and arms at sides. Slowly lift one leg off of the ground (keeping it straight) until you feel a slight pull in your hamstrings, hold for a few seconds then slowly lower it back down to starting position. Repeat with other leg keeping breathing steady throughout the movement

Standing Calf Raises

The standing calf raise is an exercise that targets the soleus muscle, which lies beneath your gastrocnemius. To do this work out, you'll need a machine with adjustable height and weight stacks (or dumbbells). You can also do this move without equipment by placing one foot on a chair or step while standing on your other leg with knees slightly bent.

Standing upright with feet firmly planted on the floor in front of you, hold onto either side of the machine's handles with palms facing inward toward each other. Inhale deeply as you lower yourself down into a squatting position by bending at both knees until thighs are almost parallel to floor; exhale as you lift yourself back up by straightening legs completely before repeating for 1-2 sets of 10-15 repetitions per leg

Machines and equipment can make these exercises easier.

- Machines and equipment can make these exercises easier.

- Machines are designed to help you perform a specific exercise with more precision, allowing for greater control of your body as well as proper technique. This can be especially helpful if you're new to working out or want a challenge that's not too difficult.

- Equipment is used to help increase resistance during workouts and make them more challenging. This can be useful if you want to build muscle mass or burn more calories than usual during one workout session (or both).

Knee Stretch

This stretch is good for the hamstrings, quadriceps and calf muscles.

- Lie on your back with knees bent and feet flat on the floor.

- Slowly straighten one leg while keeping other knee bent at 90 degrees (as shown in picture). Keep both heels firmly planted on the ground throughout this exercise. If you are stretching both legs at once, try to keep them as parallel as possible without letting them touch each other or cross over one another so that you can feel a good stretch through both hamstrings at once.

Hip Flexor Stretch

- Stand with your feet hip-width apart and knees slightly bent.

- Place one hand on a wall for support.

- Bend forward from the hips until you feel a stretch in front of your thigh; hold for 15 seconds, then repeat on opposite side.

Chest Stretch

A straightforward way to stretch your chest is by placing both hands behind your back and pulling them apart toward the ground. You can also do this while lying down on a mat, but if you have access to a machine that allows you to pull with both arms at once (such as an exercise ball or resistance band), that might be more comfortable.

If you want an extra challenge when stretching your chest muscles, try placing one hand behind each ear while doing this exercise!

Back Stretch

The back stretch is one of the easiest and most effective stretches to do. It helps to keep your spine flexible, which in turn can prevent back pain and injuries.

To perform this stretch:

- Sit on the floor with both legs straight in front of you and flat on the floor. Bend forward at the waist until your chest touches or nearly touches your thighs (but don't arch your back).

- Hold for 10 seconds on each side; repeat 5 times

Shoulder Stretch

The shoulder stretch is a great exercise for stretching your upper back and shoulders. It also helps to improve posture by strengthening the muscles that support it, and it can be done in just about any room at home or at work.

This exercise works well when performed either sitting or standing with good posture--it's important not to slouch!

Step up.

- Stand with your feet hip-width apart, holding the barbell in front of your thighs.
- Lift one foot off the floor and step up with the other foot onto a bench or box that's about knee height (you can place towels under the box if it's too high).
- Step back down with both feet and repeat for 10 reps on each side.

Step Down

- Step Down: This exercise is great for stretching the hamstrings and lower back, as well as strengthening your quadriceps muscles. It also helps to improve ankle mobility and balance.
- To perform this exercise: Stand on a step or platform with one foot, while keeping your other leg extended behind you. Slowly bend forward until you feel a stretch in your hamstrings or lower back, then hold for 30 seconds before returning to an upright position. Repeat this process with both legs (right then left) before switching to another machine or exercising machine at home!

Triceps Press down.

- Triceps Press down.

This exercise is one of the best for strengthening your triceps. The equipment you need is a weight machine, which should be available at most gyms and fitness centers. To do this exercise:

- Stand facing away from the weight machine with feet shoulder-width apart and knees slightly bent.
- Hold a barbell or dumbbells in each hand, with elbows bent at 90 degrees and palms facing forward. Lift up onto tip toes as you straighten arms to press down on both sides of upper arms (triceps) against resistance provided by the weight stacks attached to either side of your body, keeping upper arms stationary throughout movement

Shoulder Press

The shoulder press is a compound exercise that targets the deltoids and triceps.

- Stand in front of a bench, with your feet hip-width apart and knees slightly bent.

- Grab onto dumbbells with your palms facing forward and arms bent at 90 degrees by your sides (like Superman flying).

- Press both weights up until they are at shoulder height, then lower them back down to starting position. Repeat for reps (the number of times you lift the weights).

Lat Pull Down

The late pull down is a great exercise to target your lats, which are the muscles on either side of your back. To perform this exercise with proper form:

- Grasp the bar with both hands and sit with knees bent at 90 degrees and feet flat on floor or platform between legs.

- Keep back straight and chest up as you lean forward slightly toward machine's pad (or use weight stack if available).

- Keeping elbows close to sides, pull bar down until it touches upper chest; then return to start position.

Chest Press Machine

The chest press machine is an excellent way to work your chest muscles. It's not only effective, but also convenient and easy to use.

The equipment consists of two arm levers that are attached to a weight stack by cables. You sit on the seat with your feet flat on the floor and grasp one lever in each hand; then you lift them up until they reach chest level before slowly lowering them back down again. When performing this exercise, make sure that you keep good posture throughout--avoid rounding or arching your back as well as leaning forward too much (this will put unnecessary strain on your lower back).

Don't be afraid of equipment; it can be an asset to your routine.

Don't be afraid of equipment; it can be an asset to your routine.

With the right machine, you can get the same benefits as if you were doing the exercise by yourself. For example, an elliptical trainer is a great way to build up strength in your legs while also increasing cardiovascular endurance. Or try using resistance bands when weight lifting: they're easy enough for beginners but still challenging enough for advanced users!

Hip Flexor Stretch

The hip flexor stretch is a great way to stretch your inner thigh muscles and the front of your hips. To do it, stand with one foot up on a chair or bench (you can also use a wall). Bend forward at the waist and reach down toward that outstretched leg until you feel tension in your groin muscles, then return to upright position. Repeat 10 times for each side.

This exercise will help improve flexibility in these areas:

- Hip Flexors (Iliopsoas) - these are important for proper running mechanics because they help control pelvic rotation during running; if they're tight, this can lead to injury or pain when running long distances such as marathons or triathlons

Chest Opener

The chest opener is a great stretch for your chest, shoulders and upper back. To perform this stretch:

- Stand with feet shoulder-width apart and knees slightly bent.
- Place arms behind your head with palms facing forward. Pull elbows back until they are in line with ears or as far as comfortable (make sure not to lock elbow). Gently press shoulders down into a relaxed position so that chest opens up toward floor. Hold for 30 seconds on each side before moving on to next exercise or move through all four exercises in sequence two times per day

Shoulder Girdle Stretch

The shoulder girdle stretch is a great way to loosen up your upper body. It can be done without equipment, but if you have access to a stretching machine or tubing system, it's even better!

- Stand with your feet hip-width apart and hold onto the bar of a suspension trainer or other equipment that allows for easy adjustments in height (such as an Aired pad).

- With both hands in front of you on the bar, lean forward at an angle that feels comfortable for your shoulders and back--you want them snug against their respective joints. You'll know when this position has been achieved because there will be no pain in either area; rather, you should feel tension release throughout both areas as they stretch out further into their natural range of motion.

Forearm Stretch

The forearm stretch is a great exercise to help you relax and relieve tension. It's also beneficial for those who have stiff or sore muscles in their forearms, wrists, hands and fingers.

It's important to keep in mind that this stretch is not intended for everyone--if you have arthritis or other conditions affecting your joints then it may be too much of a stretch for you. If this is the case then try another type of exercise instead (see below).

Stretching can help keep you flexible, reduce injuries and improve your performance.

Stretching is a great way to improve your flexibility, reduce injuries and improve your performance.

It's important to stretch after a workout to avoid injury when you're tired. Stretching also improves circulation and helps loosen tight muscles before exercise or sports activities.

Ballet exercises

To stretch your hamstrings, use a ballet barre. This is a pole or bar that you can hold on to with one hand and step into as you bend forward at the waist.

To stretch your hips and inner thighs, stand facing the barre with feet pointed out 45 degrees from each other. Place one hand on top of the other at chest height, then slowly bend from side to side until both arms are straight down in front of you (or just slightly higher if this feels better). You may also want to try stretching one leg at a time by bringing both knees toward each other as far as possible before returning back up again slowly

Yoga has been practiced since ancient times as a way of achieving mental clarity through physical postures called asanas (posture) combined with meditation techniques such as pranayama (breathing exercises).

Strengthening exercises

Stretching and strengthening exercises are important for the health of your muscles, joints and bones. They can help you improve your balance, flexibility and strength. If you're new to exercise or have some physical limitations, it's best to start with a stretch program designed specifically for people with arthritis that is supervised by a physical therapist or other qualified healthcare professional.

The following stretching exercises can be done at home:

- Tighten all of these muscles for about 10 seconds before relaxing them again: neck muscles; shoulder blades together; arms bent at 90 degrees; elbows pointing outwards; fists clenched tightly; stomach (abdominal) muscles tightened as if trying not to laugh out loud (this will also strengthen back muscles); glutes (buttocks) tightened up so they feel like rocks under jeans!

Stretching exercises

Stretching exercises are an important part of any exercise program. Stretching often leads to better flexibility and range of motion, which can help you perform better in everyday activities as well as sports.

Stretching also helps prevent injuries by increasing the muscle's ability to resist force and lengthening muscles that have been shortened due to injury or overuse.

You should stretch before you begin any physical activity because it prepares your body for movement by increasing blood circulation, improving flexibility and warming up muscles so they don't become injured during exercise sessions. If you stretch after exercising, it allows muscles time to cool down while still maintaining their elasticity and prevents them from tightening up again quickly in response to increased demand placed on them during exercise sessions (such as running).

Exercises for the lower body

- Standing calf raise

- Squat, with or without weights

- Lunge, with or without weights

Exercises for the upper body

The following exercises can be done with the use of equipment or machines. These are a few basic moves that you can use to get started, but there are many more out there! Try researching some new stretches, and then share them with us on Facebook!

- Chest stretches: This is an excellent stretch for your chest muscles and shoulders. You'll need two chairs for this one; sit down in one chair, then lean forward so that your chest rests on top of another chair behind you (as shown). Hold for 30 seconds before repeating on other side.

- Back stretch: This stretches targets the lower back muscles by placing pressure on them from above as well as below (by bending over). To perform this exercise properly, stand straight up with feet shoulder-width apart and hands clasped behind head--then gently bend forward at waist until slight discomfort is felt in lower back area.

Exercises for the core

- Planks - A plank is a core exercise that involves lying on your belly and supporting yourself with your forearms and toes. You should keep the body straight from head to toe, with no sag in the lower back area. The key is to keep breathing and hold it for as long as possible without letting your hips drop or rise off of the floor.

- Side planks - This variation of planks requires you to support yourself on one side instead of two. Start by lying on one side with legs extended straight behind you, then lift up so that only one forearm touches down on top of the mat (similarly as if doing a push-up). Lift up into this position slowly, then lower back down slowly until both sides touch down again before repeating again!

These exercises will help you get ready to use equipment and machines at the gym.

The following exercises are meant to help you get ready for the gym and using equipment there. They should be done in order, as they build on each other.

- Toe Touch: Stand with your feet shoulder-width apart and arms straight by your sides. Bend forward at the waist until you can touch the floor with both hands and both feet. Then, slowly raise yourself back up again while keeping contact between your hands/feet and floor throughout this exercise.

- Quadriceps Stretch: Stand with one foot slightly in front of the other and bend forward at the waist until you feel a stretch in your quadriceps muscle (the large muscle group on top of each thigh). Hold this position for 15 seconds before switching legs.

The standing forward bend is an ideal stretch for lengthening your hamstrings and back.

A classic yoga pose, this exercise is great for lengthening the hamstrings and back. It also helps to improve posture by strengthening the lower back muscles.

To do this stretch: Stand with feet hip-width apart. Bend forward from your hips, reaching toward the floor with hands on thighs or fingertips on floor (depending on flexibility). If it's comfortable, move deeper into the stretch by placing hands on top of each other behind legs; if not, just stay where you are! Breathe deeply as you hold this position for 30 seconds to 1 minute before releasing slowly back into standing position

To do a standing forward bend, stand with your feet hip-width apart, then fold forward from the hips. You can also use a wall for support if you're not able to reach the floor or need extra help keeping your balance.

If you want to make it easier on yourself (and give your spine some relief), try this variation: Stand upright and bend at the waist while keeping both feet firmly planted on the floor. This is an especially good one if you have lower back pain because it stretches out those muscles without overstretching them as much as other stretches might do.

- Relax your arms and shoulders as you bend over. If you'd like, place one hand on the floor in front of you.
- Slowly lean forward until all but the backs of your legs are resting on the floor and then return to an upright position. Repeat 10 times for each leg (20 reps total).

If you can't touch your toes, that's OK. Instead, let your head hang down toward the floor but keep your back straight!

- This will stretch the hamstrings and calves.
- Make sure to keep breathing normally while doing this exercise so that you don't pass out from lack of oxygen!

Straighten up slowly when finished with the exercise, letting joints move gently as they should.

When you are finished with the exercise, straighten up slowly. Letting joints move gently as they should, keep your back straight and slowly lower your arms to the sides of your body.

Work up to holding this stretch for 60 seconds at a time; hold it anywhere between 10 and 30 seconds while practicing.

- Work up to holding this stretch for 60 seconds at a time; hold it anywhere between 10 and 30 seconds while practicing.

- If you're new to stretching, you may not be able to hold the position for very long. That is okay! As you build your flexibility, work toward increasing the time of each stretch as much as possible.

- The goal is not to feel pain but rather to feel some muscle tension without straining or forcing yourself beyond what feels comfortable in order to reach an end point (like touching your toes).

Stretching exercises are important to help people feel better after exercising or working out!

Stretching is an important part of any workout routine, but it's often overlooked. The fact is that stretching can help you feel better after exercising or working out!

If you find yourself often sore after a workout, try adding some stretching exercises into your routine. You might be surprised at how much better this makes you feel!

The best part about stretching is that it is a great way to feel better after exercising or working out. It also helps reduce the risk of injury and improve your performance. You should use stretching equipment before and after exercise, but it's also useful for warming up before intense activity. Machines can be used in addition to free weight exercises or alone if you don't have much time or flexibility but still want a great workout!

Chapter 8 – Stretching for Specific Conditions

Stretching is an important part of keeping your body healthy. If you're dealing with pain, it can help to get some "me" time to stretch out. Stretching helps relax muscles, reduces stress and tension, improves posture and alignment, increases flexibility and range of motion in joints, relieves backache, improves circulation and lymphatic flow throughout the body (which helps eliminate toxins), helps prevent injuries by increasing muscle strength and improves balance."

Ankle

Stretching the ankle is a good way to help improve your flexibility, which can help reduce pain in your feet.

- To stretch your ankles:
- Stand on one foot and lean into a wall for support if you need it. The farther away from the wall you stand, the more challenging this stretch will be (and vice versa). Keep both knees straight as you bend forward at the waist until you feel a gentle pull in the back of your leg; don't round out or hyperextend your spine during this movement! Hold this position for 10 seconds before returning to starting position and repeating on opposite side.

Back

The back is a complex structure, made up of several different muscles and other tissues. If you have back pain, stretching can help reduce it. In addition to improving your overall health and well-being, stretching can also improve posture by increasing flexibility in the spine. Stretching also helps improve breathing by increasing lung capacity and reducing stress on the body's joints.

Hamstring

The hamstring stretch is a great way to ease any tension in your lower back, hips or legs. To perform this stretch:

- Lie on your back with one leg straight and the other bent at 90 degrees.
- Bring both hands behind your head and interlace them (or just keep them together).
- Pull gently on the interlaced fingers until you feel a slight pull in the back of your thigh. Hold for 30 seconds before switching sides and repeating for two minutes total per leg.

Hip Flexors

The hip flexors are a group of muscles that attach to the front of your pelvis and thighbone. They're responsible for bringing your knee toward your chest, rotating your leg inward and stabilizing it during walking and running.

The hip flexors also play an important role in many athletic activities: they help you jump high, run fast, turn quickly and pivot on one foot without losing balance. If you have tight hip flexors (also known as "tight hamstrings"), these actions can be painful or impossible because of limited range of motion at those joints--but stretching can help improve the situation by increasing flexibility in those muscles' tendons.

Lower Back

If you work at a desk all day or spend a lot of time sitting, it can be easy to start feeling tightness in your lower back. This is because the muscles in that area are constantly being contracted as they support your spine and keep it aligned with the rest of your body. If these muscles become too tight, they pull on bones and joints which can cause pain in addition to affecting posture. Stretching can help relieve this pain by lengthening out those tight muscles so they don't pull on bones so much anymore!

Neck

If you spend a lot of time with your neck bent forward (like when you're looking at your phone), it's important to stretch the muscles in your upper back. This will help prevent muscle fatigue and pain in the neck area.

Stretching is also beneficial for people who have chronic headaches or migraines, since these pains can be caused by tense muscles in the head and shoulders.

Pectorals and Lats (chest and back muscles)

You can stretch your pectorals and lats (chest and back muscles) by lying on your back, bringing both arms over your head and grasping a towel or resistance band. Lift the towel or band up towards the ceiling and hold for five seconds before lowering it down again. You can also do this exercise with a partner by having them hold the ends of an elastic band behind their back as they stand in front of you; then reach up with both hands toward their outstretched hands while keeping elbows bent at 90 degrees.

Stretching is good for your body.

It can help to keep you flexible, reduce muscle soreness and improve circulation. Stretching can also help to reduce stress and improve mood.

The following are some examples of conditions that could benefit from specific stretches.

The following are some examples of conditions that could benefit from specific stretches:

- Joint pain and arthritis. Stretching can help to alleviate the pain caused by arthritis, especially in the hands, wrists and elbows. The key is to avoid stretching cold muscles--try doing it after warming up with some light cardio activity or a gentle stretch routine first.
- Muscle spasms. When your muscles get tight they can become over-tensed and cause painful spasms when they contract during normal use (like walking). This can lead to injuries like shin splints or runner's knee if left untreated because the body will compensate by shifting its weight around until something gives way under pressure during movement--in this case your joints! But if you're careful about stretching regularly then this shouldn't happen because it allows blood flow through those tight areas so they don't have anywhere else left but up: away from injury!

Joint Pain and Arthritis

Stretching can be a helpful way to deal with joint pain. For example, if you have arthritis in your knees and are looking for ways to relieve the discomfort and stiffness that comes with it, then stretching may be just what you need.

The following stretches are designed specifically for people who suffer from joint pain or arthritis:

Muscle Spasms

Muscle spasms are involuntary contractions of muscles. They can be painful and cause aching, tingling or numbness in the area where they occur.

Muscle spasms may be caused by:

- Lack of sleep or exercise
- Stress and anxiety

- Embarrassment or shame (for example, a muscle spasm might occur after you make an embarrassing mistake)

Plantar Fasciitis

Plantar fasciitis is a painful condition that causes pain in the heel of your foot. It's caused by inflammation of the plantar fascia, a thick band of tissue that supports your arch and connects your heel bone to your toes. Plantar fasciitis usually develops gradually over time, but it can also be brought on suddenly by strain or injury.

The symptoms include:

- Pain in the bottom of your foot when you walk or stand up after sitting for long periods (especially first thing in morning)
- Pain when going up stairs or hills

If you have these symptoms it's important for you to see a podiatrist who will examine them carefully before deciding whether treatment is necessary or not

Tennis Elbow (Lateral Epicondylitis)

Tennis elbow is a condition that causes pain and inflammation on the outer side of your elbow. It's caused by overuse of the forearm muscles. While it can be painful, tennis elbow isn't serious and usually gets better without treatment within 6 weeks to 3 months.

The exact cause of tennis elbow is unknown but it may be due to repeated stress on tendons in this area during activities such as:

- Playing tennis - hence its name!
- Playing racquet sports like badminton or squash (which can also cause golfer's elbow)

Stretching can help many people with various issues

Stretching can help you avoid pain and injury. It can also prevent surgery, if you have an issue that requires surgery. Some people who have had surgery on their knees or hips, for example, may benefit from stretching exercises to help with the recovery process.

Stretching is especially beneficial for those who are dealing with low back pain. Low back pain is commonly caused by muscle tightness in the lower back region as well as weakness in surrounding muscles (such as gluteus Medius). Stretching these muscles will help relieve tightness and improve flexibility in order to decrease any pain associated with this condition

Hip Flexor Stretch

To do the hip flexor stretch, stand with one leg behind you and your arms outstretched in front of you. Slowly lean forward until you feel a stretch in the front of that leg. Hold this position for 10-15 seconds before switching sides and repeating on the other side. You can also do this exercise by kneeling down on both knees instead of standing up straight (this will require less flexibility).

The hip flexors are responsible for bringing our legs forward when we walk or run so they play an important role in our day-to-day activities such as walking up stairs and climbing hillsides. If you have tightness in these muscles then they may not be able to move freely which could result in pain or stiffness around the pelvis area as well as lower back pain due to poor posture while walking or running outdoors/on treadmill machines at home gym equipment stores near me where I live now!

Achilles Tendonitis Stretch

The Achilles tendon connects your calf muscles to your heel bone and is one of the largest tendons in the human body. The most common cause of inflammation and pain in this area is overuse, which can lead to a condition called Achilles tendonitis. To stretch out your Achilles tendon, stand on a step with one foot and bend your other knee so that it's just off the ground. Then lean forward until you feel a stretch in your calf muscle (the large muscle behind each ankle). You can also do this stretch while sitting on the floor with both legs extended straight out in front of you--just make sure that you're sitting up straight with no bent knees!

Plantar Fasciitis Stretch

Stretching the plantar fascia is an important part of treating plantar fasciitis. The plantar fascia is a connective tissue that runs along the bottom of your foot, from your heel to just below your toes. It supports and stabilizes your arch and helps absorb shock when you walk or run.

Plantar fasciitis occurs when this tissue becomes inflamed due to overuse or injury, causing pain either in the heel or along its entire length (the sole). To stretch this area: Stand on a step with one leg straight down and bent knee on top of it; lean forward until you feel tension in both calves as well as at each end point--heel/ball/toe--of stretched limb; hold 30 seconds per stretch 3 times daily

Sciatica Stretch

If you have sciatica, a type of pain that radiates from the lower back down the back of one or both legs, stretching can help relieve your symptoms and make them less severe. Sciatica is caused by a number of different things: sometimes it's due to a herniated disc (when there is too much pressure on a spinal nerve), but it also can be due to bulging discs or degenerative disc disease.

The best way to stretch for sciatica depends on whether your pain affects only one side of your body or both sides equally. If only one side hurts when you move around in bed or sit at work, then try this exercise: Lie down on your back with knees bent and feet flat against floor; reach both arms overhead so they're parallel with ears; hold for 30 seconds before releasing slowly back down onto floor again

Low Back Pain

Stretching can be an effective way to relieve low back pain. However, it's important to understand that not all stretches are appropriate for everyone.

For example, if you have a herniated disc in your spine or broken bones in your back (such as vertebrae), it's best to avoid stretching altogether until these conditions heal. In addition, people with spinal cord injury should only do gentle stretches that don't put pressure on the spine; they should consult their doctor before starting any new exercise routine.

If you have sciatica--pain caused by irritation of one of the nerves running along our backsides--you may find that some types of stretching help ease symptoms while others make them worse. If this is the case for you, stick with gentle moves like side bends and hip flexor stretches until it seems like they're no longer aggravating things!

Plantar Fasciitis

You may be familiar with plantar fasciitis as a common cause of heel pain. It's characterized by inflammation and swelling in your foot, which can result in tenderness when you stand on your toes or walk. Plantar fasciitis is caused by overuse, obesity and high arches, flat feet and shoes that are too small or worn out.

To reduce the pain associated with this condition:

- Place a towel under the arch of your foot while sleeping to relieve stress on the plantar fascia ligament which runs across the bottom of your foot from side-to-side (front to back). This will also help distribute body weight more evenly across all parts of each foot instead of concentrating all pressure on one spot as happens when people sleep without support underneath their feet (or wear shoes without any cushioning).

Tennis Elbow aka Golfer's Elbow

Tennis elbow is a common injury that causes pain in the outer elbow. It's also called golfer's elbow, but it has nothing to do with golfing.

It's caused by repetitive bending of your wrist and forearm muscles, which put extra strain on the tendons that connect those muscles to bone. This can cause inflammation and tenderness in those tendons.

The pain usually starts gradually, gets worse over time, then goes away when you rest it for a while before returning again once you start using those muscles again (like when you pick up something heavy). The pain may be sharp or burning depending on how big an area is affected by tennis/golfer's elbow--it might radiate down into your forearm or wrist as well too!

Neck Tension and Stiffness

Neck pain is a common problem, with about 80% of people experiencing it at some point in their lives. Neck stretches can help relieve tension and stiffness in your neck, as well as improve your posture.

- Stretch your head to the side by tilting it down toward one shoulder while keeping your chin tucked slightly forward. Hold for 15 seconds and repeat on the opposite side.
- To stretch the back of your neck, tilt your head up toward the ceiling while turning from side to side as far as possible without causing any pain or discomfort (don't overstretch). You should feel this stretch

primarily along either side of where you are looking--if not, adjust so that it does! Hold each stretch for 15 seconds before switching directions again.

If you're dealing with pain, it can help to get some "me" time to stretch out.

Stretching can be a great way to relax and reduce stress. If you're dealing with pain, it can help to get some "me" time to stretch out.

Stretching helps your body feel more relaxed, which is why it's often done after exercise. It's also used as part of meditation techniques or other relaxation techniques like yoga or tai chi (a martial art).

Knee Pain

Knee pain is a common problem that can be caused by many different factors. It's often associated with overuse or injury, but it may also result from arthritis or other conditions. Poor posture can also cause knee pain, especially if you're spending long periods of time sitting down.

In most cases, you'll want to consult your doctor before starting any kind of exercise program--especially if you have chronic knee pain that hasn't responded well to other treatments like rest or medication. Your doctor will likely recommend exercises designed specifically for your condition:

- If the cause of your pain is overuse and/or injury, try strengthening the muscles around the joint using resistance bands or weights (for example). This can help prevent further injury while allowing those damaged tissues time heal properly.

If there are no signs that this type of exercise would worsen symptoms such as swelling or stiffness within 24 hours after doing them (like immediately after waking up), then feel free try these simple stretches in order help improve flexibility around tendons near joints without straining ligaments too much:

Muscle Cramps

Stretching can help prevent muscle cramps, and it also can help to alleviate them if they are already in progress. If you're experiencing a muscle cramp, try these stretches:

- To stretch the calf muscles, stand on one leg and lift your other foot behind you as far as possible while keeping both knees straight. Hold this position for 15 seconds then switch legs. Repeat 5 times per side (10 total).

- For hamstrings, bend forward at the waist with hands on thighs or calves--whatever is comfortable--and lean forward until there is no more resistance in your back muscles and hold for 15 seconds before releasing slowly back into an upright position again (this should feel like stretching all over). Repeat 5 times per side (10 total).

Stretching for Tendonitis and Bursitis

If you have tendonitis or bursitis, stretching can help relieve the symptoms and prevent these conditions from getting worse. Stretching also helps if you already have these conditions.

Here are some stretches that are especially good for helping with tendonitis and bursitis:

- Kneel on all fours with a towel under each knee so that your weight is evenly distributed across both legs. Lift one foot off the ground, keeping it straight; hold for 30 seconds before switching sides. Repeat three times per leg daily until symptoms improve (or as directed by your doctor).

- Sit on a chair with feet flat on floor or mat; use hands to press down against thighs while pulling toes back toward head until stretch feels comfortable but not painful--hold for 10 seconds before releasing slowly back into starting position

Back Pain

Stretching is a great way to help you avoid, recover from and treat back pain.

- Stretching can help you avoid back pain by keeping your muscles flexible and strong. When muscles are stiff and tight, they can pull on the joints in your spine, making them more susceptible to injury or strain.

- Stretching can help you recover from back pain by improving blood flow in the area of injury so that healing can occur more quickly than it would otherwise.

- Stretching can help you treat chronic lower-back pain simply by making it easier for them to move around without causing further damage or irritation of already sore muscles

Preventing and Treating Acute Ankle Sprains

As you've learned, stretching is an important part of preventing and treating acute ankle sprains. Stretching helps to keep your ankles healthy, flexible and strong. By performing regular stretches before activity, you can help prevent injuries by increasing blood flow to the muscles in your lower leg.

When stretching the Achilles tendon (the largest tendon in our bodies), it is important not to push yourself too far because this may cause further damage or injury. When doing any type of stretch--whether it's yoga or other physical activity--always make sure that there are no signs of pain or discomfort before continuing further with the stretch

Stretching is an important part of keeping your body healthy.

It can help to improve flexibility, which can help you avoid injury and recover quicker from an injury. Stretches also help to stretch muscles so that they don't become too tight. This can reduce the risk of muscle soreness as well as improving posture and balance.

Stretching for Back Pain

Back pain is a common condition that affects people of all ages. Stretching for back pain can help you recover from an injury, prevent further injury and feel better overall.

Back stretches are often recommended by doctors and physical therapists because they can be used to relieve muscle tension and improve flexibility in the spine. When stretching, it's important not to overstretch your muscles; instead, focus on gently lengthening them without causing pain or discomfort. To help you do this:

- Use a towel under your knees while sitting on the floor with one leg straight out in front of you (or use another object that's comfortable).
- Reach forward with both hands until they're flat against the floor; hold for 5 seconds before returning slowly into starting position--this stretch should never cause any pain!

Stretching for Foot Pain

Stretching the foot can help you avoid pain and injury. If you have foot pain, stretching your feet regularly can help to reduce or eliminate it. Stretching also helps prevent back and knee pain by improving circulation and reducing muscle tightness in these areas as well.

Stretching for Hip Pain

Stretching can be good for your body and help improve flexibility. It's important to note that stretching is not a replacement for medical treatment, but rather an adjunct to it. If you have any chronic pain or injuries, consult with a doctor before beginning any kind of exercise program.

Stretching can be especially beneficial for people who suffer from joint pain or arthritis, muscle spasms, plantar fasciitis (the painful inflammation of ligaments on the bottom of feet), tennis elbow (lateral epicondylitis).

Stretching for Neck Pain

Neck pain is a common condition that can have a significant impact on your quality of life. In fact, it's the second most common reason for seeing a doctor (after low back pain).

Stretching the neck and upper back has been shown to help reduce neck pain by increasing flexibility in those areas. It also helps with headaches caused by muscle tension or poor posture, which can contribute to or exacerbate neck problems.

To perform this stretch: Stand with feet shoulder-width apart and hands clasped behind your back. Slowly tilt head forward until you feel tension in muscles between shoulders; hold for 15 seconds or longer if comfortable; then return head upright with chin pointing straight ahead before repeating stretch three times on each side (right side first).

This can help you avoid certain types of pain.

Stretching is an important part of keeping your body healthy. It can help you avoid certain types of pain, and it's a great way to relax after a long day at work or school.

Stretching is especially useful for people who have certain conditions that cause them pain in their muscles or joints. For example, if you suffer from arthritis or fibromyalgia (a condition that causes widespread muscle pain), stretching may be able to reduce the severity of these symptoms by improving blood flow through the affected area. Stretching also helps people with chronic back pain because it increases flexibility in the spine and improves posture by strengthening muscles around joints like hips or knees which are often painful due to overuse throughout life's daily activities such as sitting at desks all day long without taking breaks throughout each hour break between classes/work shifts etcetera.

Chapter 9 – Weekly training plan

Stretching is an important part of your fitness routine. It helps keep your body limber, improves range of motion and flexibility, and can prevent injuries. There are several different types of stretching exercises, including static, dynamic and ballistic stretches. Static stretching involves holding a stretch for 30 seconds or longer while dynamic stretching uses controlled movements to increase flexibility in specific areas such as arms or legs. Ballistic stretching involves bouncing or bobbing up and down while holding the stretch position so that you're forcing the muscles beyond their normal limits for that particular movement pattern.

Warm-up:

A warm-up is an essential part of any exercise program, especially if you are new to exercise or returning from an injury. The purpose of a warm-up is to prepare the body for physical activity by increasing heart rate and blood flow to muscles, which helps prevent injury and increases performance.

A good rule of thumb for how long your warm up should be is 5-10 minutes for every 15 minutes' worth of training time (e.g., if you're going to do 30 minutes of cardio then your warm up should last at least 15 minutes). However, if you have more time available then doing an even longer warm up isn't unreasonable!

Main Sets:

- Main Sets

- Push-ups: 3 sets of 10 repetitions. Rest 1 minute between sets.

- Straight Leg Raise: 3 sets of 10 repetitions on each leg, with a 30 second rest between legs and 60 seconds total rest time between all three sets (so you'll do your left leg first, then take a 30 second break before doing your right).

Rest Periods:

Rest periods are important to allow your muscles to recover and grow. Resting 30-60 seconds between sets of each exercise is recommended, as well as taking a few minutes between exercises and workouts. It's also important to rest at least one day between days of training (e.g., Monday is chest day, so you wouldn't train again until Tuesday).

It is good for you to stretch every day, it's easy and can make a huge difference in your life.

Stretching is good for you in so many ways. It can help you avoid injury, move more easily and feel better overall. Stretching also helps to relax your body and mind, which is helpful if you're feeling tense after a long day at work or school. Stretching can even improve sleep quality by relaxing the muscles in your back and neck that are responsible for keeping our spine in alignment while we sleep.

Super Stretch

Begin in a standing position, with arms at your sides and feet slightly wider than shoulder width apart. Raise your right arm straight out to the side, palm facing forward. Bend your right elbow to 90 degrees and turn your palm toward your body as far as possible without straining or leaning forward. Rotate your torso and bring your right arm across the front of your chest as far as possible while keeping it parallel with the floor (or until it feels comfortable). Hold for 15 seconds before repeating on other side. This exercise stretches the muscles in front of our shoulders and upper back areas.

Hamstring Stretch

- Lie on your back with one leg straight and the other bent.
- Place both hands on the thigh of your straight leg and gently push it towards your chest until you feel a stretch in your hamstring (the back of your thigh). Hold for 30 seconds, then switch sides and repeat.
- Breathe deeply from nose to belly button as you hold this position for 30 seconds each time before switching sides again!

Stretches for the shoulders, upper back and spine.

Hold each stretch for 30 seconds and repeat 2-3 times. Use a towel or strap to help you with the stretches:

- Chest Stretch - Stand up straight with your feet shoulder width apart and arms at your sides. Make sure that you have good posture by keeping your chest lifted up towards the sky, shoulders back and down away from ears (not hunched forward). Bend forward from the waist until you feel a slight stretch in front of your chest muscles then hold this position for 30 seconds before returning upright again slowly rolling through each vertebra one by one as you return to standing position again maintaining good posture throughout.

Stretches for the chest, abdomen and hips.

The following stretches are designed to improve flexibility and reduce muscle tension. These stretches should be performed before your training session, as well as after each workout.

- Chest stretches: Raise your arms above your head and interlace fingers together to form a "cat stretch," keeping elbows slightly bent. Gently push into the stretch for about 20 seconds on each side of the body; repeat three times.

- Abdominal stretch: Lie flat on your back with knees bent at 90 degrees, feet flat on the floor and arms at sides (or straight out in front if it's more comfortable). Slowly raise one leg up towards the sky until you feel a gentle pull in your lower back area; hold this position for 10 seconds before lowering back down again slowly; repeat five times per side with each leg alternating between raising them up high enough so that only one foot remains on ground at all times during exercise (this helps prevent injury). You can also do this exercise while sitting upright by bending forward at waistline until elbows touch thighs then slowly raising one arm overhead while keeping other arm extended straight ahead behind body until shoulder blades meet hips--hold position for 10 seconds before switching sides (repeat 5 times per side).

Stretches for the lower back, groin and legs.

Stretching is good for your body. Stretching can help prevent injury and improve flexibility, which can lead to better posture, more energy, and an overall improved sense of well-being.

Stretching also helps with recovery from injury or surgery by reducing muscle tension and pain in the affected area(s).

Because stretching relaxes the muscles it's important for people who suffer from insomnia or poor sleep quality that stretching prior to bedtime may help them fall asleep quicker and stay asleep longer as well as reduce their morning stiffness after waking up

Do these stretches every day and you will get more flexible

So, you want to be more flexible?

Well, you're in luck! Stretching is easy and it can make a huge difference in your life. If you stretch every day, your flexibility will improve dramatically. So go ahead and try these stretches and see how much better they make you feel!

Run in place for 5-10 minutes.

Running in place is a great warm up exercise and can be done anywhere. It's also a good way to burn calories, as it raises your heart rate and gets the blood flowing through your body.

Running in place can be done at any time of day, whether it's first thing in the morning or after work when you're exhausted and want nothing more than to collapse into bed. You can even do this move while watching TV! All that matters is that you're getting those legs moving!

Cardio (20 minutes)

Cardio is the best way to burn calories and lose weight. Cardio can be done in many ways: walking, running, swimming and cycling are all forms of cardio that you can try. Cardio is also good for your heart and lungs as well as your mental health!

If you want to lose weight then doing 30 minutes of high intensity interval training (HIIT) 3 times a week will help with this goal too!

Strength training (30 minutes)

After stretching, it's important to build your strength and conditioning. This can be done through a variety of activities that focus on different muscle groups, including lifting weights and using resistance bands. Strength training is also beneficial because it improves balance and coordination, which are important factors in preventing injuries while exercising or playing sports.

Core and balance

Core and balance training is important for injury prevention, sports performance, and everyday activities.

Injury prevention: Your core muscles work together to stabilize your spine. If one part of this system isn't working properly, it can cause problems in other areas of your body. For example, if these muscles are weak or tight then they may not be able to support the spine properly which could lead to back pain or other issues such as neck pain or even headaches. This can also happen if you have poor posture which causes you strain on certain muscles while performing everyday tasks like sitting down at a desk all day long without taking breaks from sitting every hour or two minutes throughout that period of time! Sports performance: Having strong abdominal muscles will help improve speed and power output during athletic movements like sprinting across field goal lines during football games! Every day activities (like carrying groceries): Stronger abs mean less strain placed upon lower back area making it easier for someone like me who has bad knees from playing too much basketball when I was younger :)

Flexibility is important to avoid injury, improve sports performance and help you do everyday activities more comfortably.

When it comes to flexibility, most people think of stretching as an activity that only takes place in the gym or at home. But flexibility is also important on the tennis court, in dance class or even when you're doing your laundry!

Stretching is an important part of your exercise routine and should be performed before, during and after your workouts. Stretching can help you avoid injury, improve sports performance and help you do everyday activities more comfortably.

Stretching is easy to do, but it's also something that many people don't do as often as they should because they think stretching will take too much time out of their day or they're not sure how to stretch properly without hurting themselves. This is understandable--we've all been taught at some point or another that stretching before exercising could be dangerous because it would cause muscle soreness or make us weaker when we exercised later on in the day (or week). But this is not true! In fact, research has shown that proper pre-workout stretching can actually reduce muscle soreness after a workout by as much as 70%!

Monday stretching for a healthy immune system

Stretching is an important part of a healthy lifestyle. It can help you recover from illness, avoid injury, and sleep better. You may also feel more energetic after stretching!

Below are some great exercises that will help you stretch your body out on Monday morning:

Tuesday stretching for better balance and posture.

- Shoulders and upper back:

- Standing forward bend (seated if you have knee issues): Keep your arms straight and try to touch your toes with them. If this is too difficult, keep them at shoulder height and bend forward as far as possible. Breathe deeply while holding the stretch for 10 seconds. Repeat 3 times on each side.

- Chest:

- Chest stretches: Place both hands behind your back so that they are touching one another; then lift up one arm while keeping the other arm in place behind your back, stretching out through both sides of the chest at once for 30 seconds or until you feel a mild pull in that area of your body.

Wednesday stretching for increased strength and flexibility in the muscles

- Stretching is good for your muscles.

- Stretching is good for your joints.

- Stretching is good for your heart, lungs, and digestion.

- It improves circulation to the extremities and reduces swelling in the ankles and feet that can lead to circulatory problems like varicose veins or even blood clots in the legs (deep vein thrombosis).

Thursday stretching for increased cardiovascular health.

Stretching is an excellent way to improve your cardiovascular health. Stretching increases blood flow to the heart, which improves its ability to exercise. This helps you recover from exercise and reduces your risk of heart disease.

In order to stretch effectively, it's important that you understand the principles of stretching:

- Stretch slowly and gently. Don't bounce or force yourself into a stretch; instead, hold each position for about 30 seconds before moving on to the next one (or longer if needed).

- Breathe normally as you move through each stretch; don't hold your breath while stretching!

Friday:

- Stretching is important to prevent injuries.

- Stretching is good for your muscles, joints, and ligaments.

- Stretching is good for your heart and lungs.

- Stretching is good for your body's metabolism (the way it uses energy).

Stretching also helps keep the immune system strong so that you don't get sick as often!

Saturday:

- Shoulders, Upper Back and Spine:

- Chest, Abdomen and Hips:

- Lower Back, Groin & Legs:

Sunday:

- Stretching for increased strength and flexibility in the muscles

- Stretches for the shoulders, upper back and spine.

- Stretches for the chest, abdomen and hips

- Stretches for the lower back, groin and legs

- Stretch every day! It's important to stretch as often as possible, but if you are unable to do so every day, try to incorporate stretching into your routine at least three times per week. You'll be amazed at how much better your body feels and looks when it's properly stretched out!

- There are many different types of stretches: static (hold for a set amount of time), dynamic (move slowly through a range of motion), PNF (contract then relax muscle while lengthening) and proprioceptive neuromuscular facilitation (PNF). Choose one or two that work best for you based on what you're trying to achieve - strength? flexibility? balance? Try doing each type at least once per week so that all areas get worked equally well over time.

- Warm up before stretching by walking briskly around the house or yard - even if only briefly - this helps prevent injury while increasing blood flow throughout the body which allows more oxygen delivery where needed most during exercise activities later on down south later tonight ;)

CONCLUSION

In conclusion, incorporating stretching exercises into your daily routine is an excellent way for seniors to improve mobility and reduce back and joint pain. These easy exercises can be done at home in just a few minutes and provide numerous benefits for overall health and well-being. Remember to start slow and gradually increase the intensity and duration of your stretching routine. With consistency and patience, you can experience the positive effects of stretching exercises and enjoy a more active and pain-free lifestyle.

These stretching exercises for seniors are a practical and easy way to reduce back and joint pain, improve flexibility and balance, and promote overall wellness. With just a few minutes a day, you can make a significant difference in your physical health and quality of life. So why not give these exercises a try and see how much better you can feel?

Printed in Great Britain
by Amazon